The Recovery Roadmap
A Guide to Freedom and Adventure

By
Michael A. Herbert

Copyright Page

The Recovery Roadmap: A Guide to Freedom and Adventure
Written by Michael A. Herbert

Copyright © 2025 Michael A. Herbert

Published in collaboration with Voice to Book Co.

For more information on their publishing services, visit voicetobook.co or contact the team at hello@voicetobook.co.

ISBN: 979-8-89860-081-5
 Website: coachmichaelherbert.com

Table of Contents

Dedication..4

Foreword: Your Life, Your Recovery 6

Chapter One: What Recovery Really Is 8

Chapter Two: Integrity - Telling the Truth to Yourself First 18

Chapter Three: Creativity - Build a Recovery That's Yours............ 28

Chapter Four: Perseverance - Stay in Motion....................... 37

Chapter Five: Trust - Let the Process Work........................... 48

Chapter Six: Humility - The Strength to Learn from Everyone...... 58

Chapter Seven: The Three Phases of Recovery 67

Chapter Eight: When You Fall Off (And How to Get Back Up)...... 77

Chapter Nine: The Family is The Addict, The Addict is The Family, We're All in This Together.. 90

Epilogue: Fasting Forward: Embracing Imperfection on My 100-Day Journey to Clarity and Health...104

About the Author 109

Dedication

First and foremost, I wish to acknowledge my mother, Suzanne Sams, whose unwavering support has been a constant in my life through both good times and bad. She has never missed an anniversary of my recovery and has shown remarkable ability and willingness to help others in need, continuing her compassionate work well into her 80s.

To my grandmother, Beatrice Adams, whose lessons from the past have guided me toward a safer future. Her steadfast teachings have been my anchor, preventing me from falling overboard and literally saving my life through her enduring presence.

I extend my heartfelt gratitude to Robert Smith and Vince Casolaro, who entrusted me with their business, Inter Care Ltd. They provided me with opportunities to both fail and succeed in the field of addiction and recovery counseling, always recognizing my strengths and abilities. Their mentorship has been invaluable, and I would not be where I am today without their guidance.

I also dedicate this work to my brother, Van. His journey exemplifies the struggles and triumphs of recovery, reminding us that we must find what works for us to achieve success. The pain and challenges he faced have shaped him into a remarkable father, grandfather, husband, son, brother, employee, homeowner, and beekeeper.

Lastly, I wish to honor my uncle, who admired my journey but, unfortunately, could not make the same changes in his own life. He was a good person who did his best to live a meaningful life in his own way.

Foreword: Your Life, Your Recovery

I met Michael Herbert nearly two decades ago. He had just assumed the role of executive director of a "high-end" treatment center for which I'd been asked to provide clinical direction. And while years have passed since our initial encounter, I remember it as if it occurred this morning, for Michael is possessed of an indelibility of being, a presence that sticks, transcends, that simultaneously pierces and comforts. Like his voice, resonating deeply from an imposing form to provide clarity and comfort in times of need, Michael is a person who cannot and should not be easily forgotten.

While many things have changed over the last 20 years in the addiction treatment industry since Michael and I first met, the essence of Michael and his approach to recovery and life have remained consistent and deepened. During this time, many treatment centers have closed their doors, unable to survive in a hypercompetitive field for patients who can pay elevated fees for suboptimal services and luxury amenities. In contrast, Michael has thrived by becoming hyper-focused on the core principles of meaningful and lasting recovery. He continues to disdain the form while embracing the substance.

His five-step approach to recovery, outlined in this book, mirrors the essence of Michael, his approach to a meaningful life and lasting recovery. The work is clear, direct, and honest. It focuses on building an authentic life that reflects the uniqueness of every human being while simultaneously honoring the interconnectedness of all of us. Yes, it teaches us to walk in self-respect, but to do so with humility rather than hubris. In an age where success is measured by the approval and "likes" of others, Michael teaches us how to like ourselves, so we can find a place to be and to give back to a world in ways that utilize our talents to benefit others and the planet upon which we are privileged to live.

But perhaps the feature that distinguishes Michael and this work from the legions of others claiming to hold the answers to the quagmire of addictive disorders is Michael's personal journey through the brambles of his very own life. Rather than grabbing the mantle of expert, Michael assumes the role of a sherpa, a guide who knows the rocky terrain because he too has stumbled and fallen on it.

In this regard, Michael writes as a vulnerable human being who has not just fallen from grace and dignity, but who has also reclaimed his footing and scaled to higher terrain. While yes, he has had some help along the way, mainly in the form of tough love, his recovery and the value in it was derived from his efforts, by his saying "enough is enough," by stopping placing the blame for his misfortune on others, by putting on his big boy pants, and by taking personal responsibility for his actions and their consequences.

I hope you find Michael's contribution to behavioral health and addiction treatment as refreshing and valuable as I have. In a world saturated with self-proclaimed experts barking endless streams of platitudes about who and what you need to do to live a rich, meaningful and healthy life, this work stands alone. It cuts through the noise to deliver the essence of a symphony of self, a self that can emerge as a solo to join a global orchestra united in repair and resolved to share the bounty of grace with others.

Dr. Paul Hokemeyer
(J.D., PH.D)

Chapter One:
What Recovery Really Is

L et me say something that might sound strange: addiction isn't about the substance.

Yes, the drugs matter. The alcohol matters. But the real issue? It's deeper than that.

"If all I'm focused on is the substance, I'm going to miss the bigger picture and maybe relapse."

Addiction, as I've seen it in myself and in thousands of others, isn't just about what we use. It's about why we use. What we're trying to avoid. What we're trying to fill. What we're trying to feel or stop feeling.

If you strip away the crack, the alcohol, the fentanyl, the nicotine, the pills... then what's left?

For a lot of people, the answer is simple: loneliness. Emptiness. A deep sense that something's not right, not safe, not whole.

That's where addiction grows.

Beyond the Terminology

The treatment field likes to call it a "substance use disorder." And I get it. That language sounds clinical. Less loaded.

But I'll be honest: I don't love it.

"I used to like calling myself chemically dependent. That felt softer and that is what the experts called it back in the 80's. But eventually, I had to face it: I was an addict. The title did come with shame and I struggled with it. Due to my grandiosity, I also didn't want to be viewed as just an addict. My low self-esteem made me want something different. My uniqueness needed a special title, because I wasn't like 'them,' the other addicts in recovery."

Addiction, to me, is a pattern of dishonesty. Not just with other people, but with myself. It's doing something over and over that harms you, while telling yourself you're fine. It's justifying what you know deep down is wrecking your life. But it feels so good, at least for a minute.

And it shows up in more than just drugs or alcohol.

Shopping. Gambling. Cars. Sex. Food. Sugar. Power. Rage. Money. The Internet. Shoes. Property. Work. Caretaking.

Anything can become the thing we use to check out, to disappear, to escape responsibility for the pain we don't want to deal with.

And the truth is, that pain doesn't go away. Well, it does temporarily, and then it just waits and waits, and always comes back.

If you know something is hurting you or hurting the people around you and you can't or won't stop... that's something worth paying attention to.

Not because you should feel ashamed.

But because it means there's something important underneath. Something worth understanding. Something worth taking a look at. Something worth doing something about.

"You can't fix what you won't face."

The Real Numbers

Let's talk about the numbers for a second.

Roughly 10–15% of the U.S. population of 333 million people struggles with addiction at some point in their lives. Of those people, only about 10% ever receive treatment. And of those who do get treatment? Around 30% go on to maintain long-term recovery.

That means most people don't get help. And of those who do, most don't stay in recovery long-term.

That's not to discourage you.

It's to make the case that if you want a different outcome, you must engage recovery in a different way.

Not as a 30-day fix. Not as punishment. Not because someone else is making you.

But because you want to change. Because you want more. And even if the more is just comfort, you've got to make a change.

And if you're willing to face the truth about your patterns, your pain, and your power, change can happen.

The First Nine to Eighteen Months Are Discovery, Not Recovery

There's a big difference between stopping and being in recovery.

Abstinence is about stopping the use. Recovery is about changing the relationship you have with yourself. Learning to love yourself takes time, it takes years. So don't pick up if it doesn't happen right away. The goal is to stay clean no matter what. Time and action will take care of the rest.

"When I stopped using, that was just the start. The real work was rebuilding the life underneath it."

I always tell people the first nine months aren't recovery; they're discovery. That's when you're just starting to figure out who you are without the substance. You're learning what triggers you. You're uncovering the patterns that brought you here in the first place.

It's messy. It's confusing. And sometimes it feels worse before it feels better.

When I first got into recovery, I wasn't ready for a lot of it. People suggested all kinds of things: get a sponsor, work the steps, go to therapy, change everything in your life.

For some of that, I wasn't ready. And that's okay.

What I knew for sure was that I needed to stop. I needed abstinence. Without that clarity, I couldn't even begin to figure out what else I needed.

But abstinence alone wasn't enough. I had to start discovering who I was, what worked for me, and what didn't work.

I didn't know who I was without the chaos. I'd been using for so long that drugs had become my solution for everything: stress, boredom, celebration, pain, connection, isolation. When I stopped, I had to learn everything all over again along with some new things.

That's why I call it discovery. You're discovering what triggers you. What calms you. What gives you purpose. What helps you stay clean one more day.

You're discovering what you need physically: better food, more movement, actual sleep. You're discovering what you need mentally: new thoughts, new tools, new support. You're discovering what you need emotionally: connection, expression, understanding. You're discovering what you need spiritually (not religiously): connection, creativity, trust, serenity.

And all of that takes time. More than 30 days. More than 90 days. More than a year.

"They say it takes 5 years of being clean to get your brains back. And another 5 years to learn how to use them." - Anonymous

The Family Has an Addiction Problem

Here's something else I've learned over the years: addiction isn't just a problem for the person using. It's also a family problem.

The addict is the family. And the family is the addict. The addict is a part of the family, and the addiction is pulling the strings for everyone.

People sometimes want to separate the addict from everyone else, as if they're the only one with the problem. But addiction affects the entire system. Everyone around the addict starts to change their behavior, their expectations, their hopes, their boundaries.

The wife, the husband, the son, the daughter of the addict all experience the same consequences of the addiction: concentration problems, eating too much, eating too little, headaches, stress sensitivity, slips and falls, intimacy problems, poor boundaries, isolation, money problems, health problems, fear, anger, self-pity, negative thinking, hopelessness—the list goes on. The same negative experiences as a result of the addiction.

Everyone in the family system gets caught up in the chaos. They start enabling, controlling, rescuing, avoiding, denying. They develop their own unhealthy patterns to cope with the unpredictability and instability of addiction.

They need help too. Sometimes even more than the addict.

I've worked with family members who pay the rent, the car note, their drug dealers, the phone bill and the cigarettes for their addicted loved one who's in rehab. They're still being affected by addiction. "I have to pay their rent while they're in rehab, or they will lose their apartment," is what they think. "I have to make sure they have a place to go when they get out."

When do you start to recover from feeling responsible for doing for someone what they should do for themselves? When do you focus on your own well-being?

Recovery is for the whole unit. Not just the individual. Because everyone has been affected by addiction.

Let me give you an example. I worked with a family where the father was sending his son to one rehab after another. Ten years, nearly half a million dollars, and the son was still getting high.

The father was obsessed with fixing his son. He couldn't sleep, couldn't focus at work, couldn't enjoy any part of his life because he was constantly worrying about his son.

When I started working with them, I told the father a hard truth: "You're as addicted as your son. He's addicted to drugs. You're addicted to saving him."

It took time for him to see it. But eventually, he realized that his constantly rescuing his son wasn't helping either of them. It was in fact keeping them both stuck.

When he started to work on his own recovery—setting boundaries, focusing on his own well-being, letting his son face the consequences of his choices—everything started to shift. The son actually had to confront his addiction without his father swooping in to clean up the mess. And the father started to find peace again, regardless of what his son chose to do.

The father moved from enabling the disease of addiction, to enabling recovery. And when the father changed, it forced his son to change.

Beyond Abstinence

Recovery, real recovery, is about so much more than just not using.

I see a lot of people making the same mistake. They think if they can just stop drinking, stop using, stop gambling, then everything will be fine. And sometimes they do manage to stop for a while. But they don't change anything else about their lives.

They're still the same person with the same patterns, the same triggers, the same void they're trying to fill. They're just trying to "white-knuckle it" without their solution.

That's not recovery. That's abstinence. And while abstinence is essential, you can't recover with just abstinence. It's not sufficient. Just abstinence from drugs and alcohol leads you into filling that hole with something else. Work. Food. Sex. Gambling. Power. You name it, and none of them are good. They say workaholism is the only disease they applaud.

Real recovery is about rebuilding your life in a way that supports staying clean. It's about addressing the underlying issues that drove you to use in the first place. It's about developing new coping skills, new relationships, new ways of thinking.

It's about changing your relationship with yourself.

For me, that meant finding new ways to challenge myself: climbing mountains, running ultra-marathons, traveling to places I'd only dreamed of. It meant eating better, moving more, sleeping enough. It meant learning to meditate, to journal, to talk honestly about what I was feeling. And it was also about going to the doctors and the dentist for check-ups. Maybe I could get back that million-dollar smile—anything would be better than a back-alley five-dollar grin. (jk)

It meant finding a purpose bigger than myself, whether that was helping others in recovery or supporting children's education in Ethiopia.

And it meant doing all of this in my own way, finding what worked for me, even if it didn't look like anyone else's recovery.

That's what I want for you: a recovery that's uniquely yours. A recovery that's sustainable. A recovery that's worth staying for.

Not because someone else says you should.

But because you've built a fulfilling life that you don't want to lose.

Reflection

Take a moment to consider:

1. What have you been focusing on in your recovery so far? Just stopping the behavior, or building something new?

2. Who in your life has been affected by your addiction? How might they need recovery too?

3. What's one small thing you could do today to move beyond abstinence and into true recovery?

Remember, this isn't about getting it perfect. It's about starting where you are and taking one step forward.

You don't need to have all the answers right now. You just need to be willing to ask the questions.

Chapter Two:
Integrity – Telling the Truth to Yourself First

I once had a client—I'll call him Marcus—who sat across from me in session, arms folded, mouth tight, eyes darting toward the exit every few minutes like he was planning a jailbreak.

He'd been sent to me by his job. Failed a drug test, claimed it was a "false positive," and said he didn't need treatment, he just needed to "check the box" and get back to work.

You could feel the defensiveness rolling off of him.

I let him talk. Let him posture. I wasn't there to argue.

At some point, I asked him, "Let's say the test was wrong. Why do you think they assumed it wasn't?"

He went quiet.

Then, slowly, he said, "Because they don't trust me."

I nodded. "Why do you think that?"

He said: "I don't know."

I said: "Well, what if you did know?"

More silence. But this silence was the real kind—the kind where you could tell something was clicking into place.

A week later, Marcus came back. He looked different. A little more grounded. And he said something I've never forgotten:

"It's not just that they don't trust me. It's that I don't trust myself. I lie so easily now, I don't even notice I'm doing it."

That moment? That was the beginning of his recovery.

What Integrity Means in Recovery

People talk about integrity like it's this big, noble thing—like honesty put up on a pedestal. But in recovery, integrity isn't always dramatic. It's in the small decisions. The tiny forks in the road. The quiet moments when no one's watching and you ask yourself: Am I being real right now?

When I was in active addiction, I had no integrity. Not because I was a bad person. But because I couldn't afford to be honest.

Honesty required facing reality, and reality was the one thing I couldn't handle.

So I lied. To others. To myself. I minimized. I shifted blame. I would tell myself this is just temporary, or everyone does it, or at least I'm not as bad as the other guy.

But integrity is allergic to excuses.

"Integrity is doing what's right, even when it's hard, even when no one's clapping, even when the only one who'll know is you."

That's not easy. Especially early on. Especially when shame still has you in a headlock. And ego is running the show.

But here's the thing: integrity isn't about being perfect. It's about being willing to tell the truth, even when it's inconvenient.

It's calling your therapist back when you said you would. It's showing up for your group when you feel like shit. It's admitting when you screwed up instead of hiding it or spinning it into something it wasn't.

It's not some grand gesture. It's a practice.

The Cost of Dishonesty

One of the sneakiest ways we lose integrity in recovery is by trying to present as recovered. We want people to think we're okay. We want to feel okay. So we fake it.

And that works... until it doesn't.

Because faking it is exhausting. And eventually, it collapses under its own weight.

So let me say this plainly: you don't have to have it all together.

You just have to be honest about where you're at.

If you're struggling, tell someone you're struggling. If you're scared, say that you're scared. If you're not sure what you believe, or what you want, or who you might be without the chaos, express that uncertainty.

That's integrity.

Many think that recovery is about simply stopping the behavior. But real recovery? It's about rebuilding trust—with yourself first, and others later.

And trust starts with truth.

"When I lie—even a little—I create distance between who I am and who I say I am. That gap is where addiction sneaks back in."

Integrity closes that gap.

It's the daily, sometimes hourly, act of choosing alignment over avoidance. Truth over image. Responsibility over comfort.

Not because you have to, but because you want to live a life that truly feels like your own.

My Ethiopia Story

Let me tell you a story about integrity that changed my life.

I was in Ethiopia, waiting for another group to join us in the Dalol area, which is the hottest place on earth. I met the village leader, who showed me his small village. The school and the village had been blown over and destroyed by a dust storm. This village was in the middle of the desert. Nothing grows there. It is so hot that these children, along with their parents and grandparents, will never experience a glass of ice water in their lifetime. Something I take for granted.

I told the man, "If I ever come back, I'll bring some school supplies." It was just one of those things you say, a nice gesture, but I didn't think much more about it at the time.

By September of that year, I was looking at my pictures again and thought, "I've got to go back to Ethiopia." Then I remembered my promise about the school supplies. Now what am I going to do?

I decided to do a fundraiser, planning to raise about $1,800 for some pens, pencils, and other basic supplies. Within a week, I had raised $3,000. Shortly after that, more than $20,000.

I created a non-profit called African Hopeful Horizons to maximize the potential of these resources, because I wasn't going to bring $20,000 worth of pens and pencils. On my first trip back, I took nine suitcases filled with pens, pencils, notebooks, solar calculators—anything I could bring. I was also fortunate enough to obtain a donation of school supplies from Office Depot, and Peter Glen Ski Shop provided t-shirts for all of the students. I was able to supply that school and two other schools with a year's worth of educational materials.

The following June, I made another trip back, bringing more supplies to one particular school. I realized that the kids also needed lunch each day, so a sustainable solution popped in my head: "Chickens!" I said, "If you can build a chicken coop, I'll provide the chickens." They built the coop, and I put up the roof and installed the windows, and then filled it with 53 chickens from an Ethiopian chicken farm to start.

I flew in a woman who owned a restaurant in Addis Ababa (who also happened to be an ally for people in recovery) to Tigray region to oversee the project. We then had 53 chickens producing eggs for the children's lunch program. That was the start. We now also have 150 reproducing chickens so that we are able to provide lunch for the students five days a week. And then having the ability to pay for the chicken food, and upkeep, and they built a second chicken coop.

We've also cemented all the school floors so they're not walking on dirt. We cemented the walls, fixed the windows, and provided desks for 127 students. Every child has a book bag, calculator, pens—things they wouldn't have if we hadn't helped.

Why am I telling you this story? Because it's about more than charity. It's about integrity—keeping a promise that could have been easily forgotten or ignored. It's about following through, even when it would have been easier not to.

In recovery, we often make promises to ourselves and others. "I'll change." "I'll do better." "I'll be there for you." "I'll show up differently this time." And then we don't follow through. We let ourselves off the hook. We make excuses. We justify our inaction.

But integrity demands that we keep our promises, both to others and to ourselves. Even the small ones. Especially the small ones. Because that's how trust is rebuilt. That's how we close the gap between who we say we are and who we actually are.

And sometimes, keeping one small promise leads to something much bigger than you could have imagined.

When Others Won't Tell the Truth

Integrity isn't merely a personal virtue; it's a reflection of the systems around us, the very fabric woven by the people who are meant to support us, and the standards to which we hold one another. It is in these moments of truth that we reveal our true character or lack thereof.

I once was working with a client who happened to be a primary therapist working within a treatment program. While this person was providing individual therapy, facilitating groups and working with families, they were secretly engaged in their own addiction. They were hiding their drug use from their peers and the clients. When the facade crumbled, and the secret came out, they were removed from their position as a therapist, but compassionately offered support to seek treatment for their addiction. However, the very program that was tasked with guiding her towards recovery failed to impose the critical guard rails and accountability measures to keep her from returning to work as a therapist prematurely. They inexplicably encouraged her to continue working with mentally ill patients, all the while advising against involvement with those struggling specifically with Substance Use Disorders.

This individual was not reported to any regulatory board. The only recommendations made for her were a thirty-day treatment program, a halfway house, and ongoing therapy. Yet, therein lay the crux of the issue: there were no mandates, no accountability. This person was never required to demonstrate the ability to maintain abstinence for even the barest minimum of time before re-entering the field, regardless of it being general Mental Health or Substance Abuse. And I believe for a therapist to resume practice, the required bare minimum period of abstinence from using drugs is one year after a therapist returns to using drugs from a period of abstinence. In addition, I don't consider this a relapse as I question if this person was actually ever in what I would consider recovery.

But they did achieve abstinence, got their master's degree legitimately, and was able to work in the field of addiction. As history would predictably reveal, within a mere sixty days of purported abstinence, they resumed working with clients. The tragic cycle began again: they fell back into substance use, spiraling downward while masquerading as a helper to others. This is an example of the return to substance abuse without any real treatment of addiction or demonstration of change other than what I would call superficial compliance.

To make matters worse, this person even secured a glowing recommendation from their mental health supervisor at the university they attended. The former employer, the rehabilitation center, and the university professor all had the opportunity to intervene, to uphold integrity, yet each chose to enable her addiction. What a profound disservice to her and to the entire industry.

When I finally sat down with her, I had to deliver an unvarnished truth: "Your behavior poses a danger not only to yourself but to those you claim to help. I have a duty to protect the integrity of this industry along with my own integrity and beliefs. Your judgment is impaired by your addiction and substance use; you should not be working with vulnerable individuals at this time."

I laid out the stark choices before her: "You must step away from your practice. Your mind is clouded, and addiction is steering your life. When you are using, preoccupied with the thought of using, or managing the aftermath of your using, you cannot reliably help others. You are certainly not helping yourself."

Anger surged within me, not directed at the client, who was clearly unwell, but at the institutions, the individuals, and the disease of addiction that had enabled this destructive cycle. They had turned a blind eye, prioritizing reputation and convenience over integrity, and in doing so, had betrayed not just her but the very principles our profession stands upon.

Sometimes, integrity demands solitude. It requires us to take unpopular stands, to act with conviction in the face of collective complacency. We might even call that courage.

But this is the essence of recovery: not perfection, but raw honesty, even when the truth is hard to bear. Especially when it's hard.

Reflection & Practice

Integrity in recovery isn't something you achieve once and for all. It's something you practice daily, in small moments and big ones.

Here are some questions to consider:

1. What's one area of your life where you're not being completely honest—with yourself or others?

2. What would it look like to practice integrity in that area this week?

3. How do you respond when someone calls you out or when you catch yourself in a lie?

4. Think about a time when you did choose integrity, even when it was hard. What came from that choice?

Remember, integrity isn't about being perfect. It's about being willing to tell the truth, even when it's uncomfortable. It's about closing the gap between who you are and who you say you are.

Start small. Be honest about one thing today that you might normally hide or minimize. See how it feels. See what opens up when you choose truth over comfort.

The path of integrity isn't always easy. But it's the only path that leads to real recovery.

Chapter Three:
Creativity - Build a Recovery That's Yours

Recovery isn't just about removing something. It's about creating something.

If you're not careful, recovery can start to feel like a list of do's and don'ts. Don't use. Don't lie. Don't get into a relationship. Go to 90 meetings in 90 days. Get a sponsor. Stay away from people, places and things. And while those boundaries matter, they're not enough to build a life you actually want to live.

"I didn't get into recovery to be good. I got into recovery to be free."

This is where creativity comes in. Not artistic talent or paint-on-a-canvas creativity, but the kind that lets you imagine something new. Something that fits who you are, not who someone else tells you to be.

Early on, I realized I wasn't going to make it if I didn't find ways to stay curious, challenged, and connected to something bigger than just "not using."

So, I started doing things that would enhance my recovery experience. Just going to work, meetings and therapy wasn't enough.

I took a primitive living course. I started running. I became a beekeeper. I traveled. I started CrossFit. I took an acting class. I climbed mountains.

Over time, based on my athletic ability, I began to identify myself as a professional athlete. Not needing permission from anyone else, I worked so hard for that title and took ownership of that title. Not needing anyone else's approval to be what I had worked for.

"My recovery couldn't be built around what I wasn't doing. It had to be built around what I was creating."

Finding Your Own Path

There's a moment from a hike that I'll never forget. Not just because it was hard, but because of what it revealed.

I was climbing Mount Meru in Tanzania. I thought I'd be the strongest one in the hiking group, but I quickly realized that I wasn't. I was in fact the slowest. I'm not sure if it was due to jet lag, altitude, or improper training, but I was last at every rest stop. At every stretch, I struggled. But I just kept going.

The irony? I had asked to hike alone, worried that others would slow me down. As it turned out, I was the one who needed more time.

And I needed to be honest about my limits. Adjusting my story. Letting go of what I thought it should look like.

It's not about being impressive. It's about staying in motion, even if the motion is slow motion.

In recovery, we often get caught up in doing it "right." We think there's a formula, a perfect path, a set of rules that, if followed exactly, will guarantee our success.

But what if that's not true?

What if recovery is more about discovering what works for you, even if it's different from what works for everyone else?

Another thing I realized in my time in recovery is that those before me and around me often talked about the ideal and I'd compare their ideal with what I was doing. I realized later that anytime I compare myself with anyone, someone's got to lose, and for a long time it was me. Again, my recovery is taking responsibility for me.

This doesn't mean ignoring the wisdom of those who have gone before me. It means taking what works and leaving what doesn't. It means being willing to experiment, to try new things, to build a recovery that actually fits my life.

For me, that meant adventure. It meant pushing my physical limits. It meant exploring the world. It meant challenging myself in ways that had nothing to do with drugs or alcohol.

What might it mean for you?

The Hyena Story

This might be a good place to talk about the hyena.

Hyenas get a bad rap. People think they're scary, can't be trusted, gross or just nature's cleanup crew. But here's the truth: hyenas are some of the most resilient, resourceful, and intelligent animals in the wild.

They survive because they adapt. They work in a community. They find ways to thrive in harsh conditions and they don't need anyone else's approval to do it.

"I used to feel like a hyena—misunderstood, underestimated, looked down upon and on the outside. But the more I learned about them, the more I saw myself."

When I think of my recovery process, I think of hyenas because hyenas have this perseverance where they're not the fastest, but they will run down an animal until they get it. They will wear that animal out so they can get fed, so they can get a meal. There's just something about that consistency, just kind of trotting, doing the best you can. It's kind of like the tortoise and the hare—how the tortoise just kept going. He wasn't the fastest, but he was consistent in moving forward. And he eventually won the race.

In Ethiopia, I visited Harar, a village where wild hyenas roam like stray dogs. This is a place where you can actually feed them. You sit on a log, wrap a piece of meat on a stick, and hold it in your mouth. The hyena comes and takes it right from you.

I've felt those hyenas bump against me. You can feel the power of that animal. You hear their distinctive laughing call. There's fear that comes up around hyenas, but they're just trying to eat and take care of their families.

That's recovery, too. It's about finding your own way, even when others don't understand it. It's about persevering when the path gets hard. It's about using your intelligence, your resources, your community to survive and eventually, to thrive.

You don't need to be a lion.

You just need to be you.

When No One Else Is Doing What You Need

Recovery isn't a solo journey. But sometimes, the path you need to take is one that others aren't walking.

I remember starting my discovery process. They pushed me towards attending the alcohol fellowship. There weren't people who looked like me there. Many of them were older white men, and as a 29-year-old black man, I didn't think I could relate. I did find an alternative fellowship where the people looked more like me, closer in age, and in a place where I felt comfortable. Back then I needed that comfort in order to help get the message. This was just a simple change that I made, I took responsibility for my recovery, I didn't quit, I just adjusted my program as I found something that worked for me.

Many years later I found myself in a situation while living in Egypt. The only English-speaking fellowship to attend was like the alcohol-focused group back home, where I originally did not relate to. However, by this time I was 16 years in recovery and had made changes in my thoughts and attitudes. Being many years older, I was able to set aside my differences. I did still believe in the possibility of getting my needs met at a deeper level. I knew my heart was in this new fellowship. So, with some help from others, with that fellowship we were able to start the first English-speaking 12-step alternative fellowship in Egypt. That was back in 2005. That meeting is still going on today.

Sometimes what we need may not be out there. And if it's not, maybe it is our responsibility to create it.

I experienced this again when I wanted to connect with other black men on a deeper, more intimate level and I didn't believe that a 12-step fellowship was enough. I also didn't want that hierarchy of having a therapist-led group. So, what happens when you want something that's not available? Your job is to create it.

I started a black men's journal group where we meet and share our intimate thoughts and feelings about how we feel as men, how we feel as black men; our self-esteem, employment, value, sex, purpose in life, relationships, spirituality—all these things that there isn't often a safe place to talk about.

We meet for an hour and a half twice a month and talk about what we write in our journals, how we feel. We're open to feedback from each other. We also engage in meditation at the beginning of the group and end with a prayer.

It's an opportunity for us to level with each other, to share on a deep emotional basis, to confront things we don't particularly want to confront. Infidelity is a big topic that comes up. So is self-esteem and self-worth. Asking for money is another—most of us haven't learned how to ask for what we're worth or what we need.

The group includes people across the socioeconomic spectrum. We all need that safe space to be honest, to be vulnerable, to be seen.

Creating What Isn't There

Creativity in recovery means asking: What makes me feel alive? What can I build instead of break? What's something I've always wanted to try, but never let myself?

It could be painting. It could be hiking. Could be cooking, parenting, designing, writing, singing, sailing, beekeeping, boxing, learning Portuguese, mentoring kids, or going back to school.

Whatever it is, it's yours.

Don't wait for someone else to give you permission. Don't worry if it doesn't look like anyone else's path.

You're not here to impress anyone. You're here to build something that keeps you coming back.

I remember reading a GQ Magazine article in the early nineties. It was about a survival school in the deserts of Utah. It fascinated me. I showed my boss and said, "Hey, Bob, what do you think about this? These people are living in the desert of Utah and just surviving. Boy, this really seems interesting."

He said to me, "Why don't you do it?"

I had never thought to actually do it. I only thought to daydream about it. But his question sparked something in me. I called the Boulder Outdoor Survival School and signed up for the course.

I wound up in the desert of Utah doing my first survival school. I thought, "Wow, what an adventure, what a learning experience." The only goal was food, water, and shelter. We walked around the desert looking for these basic necessities. It was one of the best experiences of my life.

That's how creativity works in recovery. You think about something you've always wanted to do. And instead of just thinking about it, you actually do it.

It might seem weird—climbing a mountain, running 155 miles through the Sahara Desert, taking a primitive living course and living with the Tarahumara Indians, or climbing an active volcano, or even feeding wild hyenas. These trips are very inconvenient at times. You're filthy, you're dirty. There's no soft bed to sleep on, or a decent place to go to the bathroom. And I'm spending money to do it!

But these experiences change my life. They challenge me physically. They introduced me to amazing people. They give me memories that sustain me through difficult times.

These are the things that I wanted to do. I couldn't get a whole bunch of people to sign up and do them with me, so I signed up, took the risk and went out on my own.

They helped me build a life worth living.

Reflection & Practice

Creativity in recovery isn't about being artistic—it's about building something new. Something that's uniquely yours.

Here are some questions to consider:

1. What brings you energy, even if you've been told it's not practical or important?

2. Are you following someone else's idea of what recovery "should" look like?

3. What's one creative risk you're willing to take in your recovery this month?

4. If you gave yourself permission to start something new, what would it be?

Recovery isn't just about stopping something destructive. It's about starting something constructive. Something that excites you. Something that challenges you. Something that makes you want to get up in the morning.

You don't have to know exactly what that is yet. You simply must be willing to explore. To try things. To see what fits.

The most beautiful recoveries I've seen aren't the ones that follow some perfect formula. They're the ones that reflect the uniqueness of the person living them.

So what will yours look like?

Let yourself imagine.

Chapter Four:
Perseverance – Stay in Motion

There's a lot of talk in recovery about surrender. Letting go. Accepting powerlessness. Trusting the process. Yes, those things matter. Faith moves mountains, but you should bring a shovel.

Because sometimes, what you really need is to dig in.

There will be days when everything in you wants to quit. When the old life calls out like a siren. When the new life feels too far away.

Perseverance is what keeps you moving.

Don't let lack of motivation stop you; motivation isn't necessary. I find it works the opposite, doing the work gets me motivated not the other way around.

Let me be clear: I didn't get here because I made one big decision and stuck to it perfectly.

I got here because I made small decisions over and over again.

I tried to quit smoking six or seven times before it stuck. That doesn't mean I failed six times. It means I kept coming back.

"Perseverance isn't about getting it right. It's about getting back up—again and again—until something shifts."

People sometimes ask me how I've stayed in recovery so long.

I say, "Because I never gave up. Even when I wanted to."

That might sound simple. It's not.

There were times I thought about getting high again. Times I thought about disappearing. Times I thought, what's the point of all this?

But then I'd go for a run. Or I'd put pen to paper. Or I'd call someone I trusted. Or I'd remind myself of what it felt like at my lowest—cold, hungry, alone, staring into a store window at a version of myself I didn't recognize.

And I'd think: Not today.

Just not today.

That's how you build a recovery that lasts.

Not by being the strongest. Not by never messing up.

But by staying in the game.

Even when you're tired.

Even when you're not sure it's working.

Even when it would be easier to go numb.

"There's no finish line. Just the next right step."

The Marathon Through the Sahara

I want to tell you about the most physically demanding thing I've ever done—running 155 miles through the Sahara Desert.

Picture this: 110-degree heat. Sand everywhere. A marathon a day for four days, then 58 miles on the fifth day.

Of about 180 people who started that race, only 117 finished. I finished at 114 out of those 117—the fourth slowest person to complete the race.

But here's my claim to fame: I beat the youngest guy, who was 19 years old.

I was in my fifties. Two hundred and thirty pounds. Running through the Sahara Desert.

After the first 18 miles, my feet swelled up so much that I could no longer wear my running shoes. So, for the next 137 miles I ran my race in a pair of Tevas.

It was a miracle that I completed it, but I did.

About 5 miles before the end of the race, I could see the finish line. And I said to myself, "You know what Michael, why don't you just quit right now?" And as I said that a woman who was also in the race came up behind me. She looked just as tired and exhausted as I was. But what I noticed was that she didn't have any shoes on and was running in her socks. She told me she had to ditch her shoes about a mile ago and was going to complete the race in just her socks.

And at that moment I said, "If she can do it, I can do it," and I continued on. One of the things that happens in recovery is that you get these moments of sanity. These opportunities to rethink your decisions. That was such an opportunity for me. And you will get them too.

There will be times when you want to use, you'll be ready to use and something will happen, and you'll get an opportunity to change your mind. And you must grab on to that. Because oftentimes it's just a moment, just a second. And grabbing that moment or second can save the day.

Another experience I had during that race was at night. Everyone had to wear a light on their back so you could see the person in front of you, and the person behind you could see you. We followed each other through the darkness.

That's what recovery is like. I need to follow the person who's a few steps, a few feet, a few weeks, or a few years ahead of me. And I also need to be leading someone else in that process.

I'm responsible for helping someone, and I'm also responsible for getting help from someone else.

Both of those things are essential to making it through.

During that race, I learned something about perseverance that I'll never forget. It wasn't about being the fastest. It wasn't about looking good. It was about keeping going, one step at a time, no matter how slow or how difficult.

There was only going to be one winner anyway. The rest of us were just trying to finish. And finishing was enough. More than enough.

For me it was about completing, not competing.

That's true in recovery, too. It's not about doing it perfectly or impressing anyone. It's about moving forward, a step at a time, as you engage in that never-ending finish line.

Getting Back Up (Again and Again)

When I talk about perseverance in recovery, I'm not just talking about the big, dramatic moments. I'm talking about the everyday decision to keep going.

The decision to get out of bed when depression is telling you to stay there.

The decision to call someone when shame is telling you to isolate.

The decision to tell the truth when fear is telling you to hide.

These small acts of perseverance add up. They build a foundation for your recovery that can withstand the storms that will inevitably come.

Because here's the thing: recovery isn't a straight line. It's not a steady climb upward. It's a series of ups and downs, forwards and backwards, moments of clarity and moments of confusion.

The key isn't to avoid the downs. The key is to keep getting back up.

I remember when I was first trying to get clean. I'd make it a few days, then slip. Make it a week, then slip. Each time, the voice in my head would get louder: "See? You can't do this. You're not strong enough. You're not good enough. Just give up."

But something in me refused to believe that. Something in me knew there was more to my story than just failure.

So, I kept trying. Kept reaching out. Kept showing up to meetings even when I didn't want to. Kept calling people and talking even when I was embarrassed. Kept telling the truth even when it hurt. And when talking about it when it was too hard to talk about, I put pen to paper.

And slowly, inch by inch, day by day, I built a recovery that stuck.

Not because I was special. But because I was stubborn. Because I refused to let addiction have the last word in my story.

You can do the same. It doesn't matter how many times you've tried before. It doesn't matter how many times you've slipped up. What matters is that you keep getting back up.

Keep trying. Keep reaching out. Keep showing up.

That's perseverance. And it's the heart of recovery.

The only time you don't get back up is when you're in the ring with Mike Tyson and he punches you in the face. When he knocks you down, you surrender. Just like we talk about in recovery. It's ok to surrender in recovery and give up the fight to find a new way to live.

Finding Your Payday

One of the most important aspects of perseverance in recovery is finding your "payday." What do I mean by that? I mean finding what makes all the hard work worth it. Finding what gives you the ability to keep going, even when it's difficult.

Because let's be honest: recovery is hard work. It's uncomfortable. It's challenging. It asks you to face the things you've been running from. It asks you to feel the feelings you've been numbing. It asks you to change patterns that have been with you for years, maybe decades.

If there was no payoff for that work, why would you do it?

When I was first getting clean, I had to find my payday. I had to find what made staying clean more important than using. I had to find what made the work of recovery worth it.

For me, that payday came in many forms. It came in the form of physical health—being able to run, to climb, to move my body in ways that felt good. It came in the form of mental clarity—being able to think clearly, to make decisions, to solve problems. It came from getting a job that I liked. That paid me enough to be able to live in this new way of life. It came in the form of relationships—being able to connect with others and to build trust.

But it also came in the form of adventure—being able to travel, to explore, to push my limits in ways I never thought possible.

That's what kept me going. That's what made the hard work worth it.

What's your payday? What makes the work of recovery worth it for you?

Maybe it's your children. Maybe it's your career. Maybe it's your physical health. Maybe it's your spiritual connection. Maybe it's losing weight, maybe it's gaining weight. Or maybe it's the dream of a life you've always wanted but never thought you could have.

Whatever it is, hold onto it. Remind yourself of it when the going gets tough. Let it pull you forward when you feel like giving up.

Because when staying clean becomes more important than getting high, that's when recovery sticks. When you can find a payday for the work that you do, that's when you commit to the work.

Find your payday. And let it fuel your perseverance.

When Your Body Says "Enough"

There's a story I want to share with you about perseverance, but also about knowing your limits.

I recently climbed Mount Meru in Tanzania. It was one of the most physically demanding experiences I've ever had. This mountain was relentless—up, up, up all the way. There were no plateaus, no breaks.

I had done Kilimanjaro two years before, and Machu Picchu before that. I thought I was ready. In fact, I told the guide, "Make sure I go on this by myself because I don't want anybody slowing me down."

But when I showed up, there were six other people waiting to go up with me. It turned out they all had more experience than I did. Two women from Switzerland who climbed the Swiss Alps all the time. A younger woman from Poland who seemed to have climbed every mountain on earth. Two women from

44

Norway who climbed regularly. And a couple from Indonesia who were mountain guides.

I was the least experienced. And at every rest stop, I was the last person to arrive. I got the least amount of rest because everyone had to wait for me, and then it was time to go again.

One day we hiked for five hours. Another day it was eight hours. And then after that eight-hour hike, we were supposed to rest for about six hours before summiting at midnight.

But I told the guide, "I'm done. I cannot summit. I can't take another step up this mountain."

This was the first time my body talked to me and told me, "Michael, you've gone as far as you can go." Usually, it's my mind that tells me I can go further or that I should stop. But this time, it was my body.

And in that moment of telling the guide I wasn't going further, I didn't tell myself, "Michael, you're a failure. You should do it anyway." What I focused on was the journey up the mountain. As hard as it was, how challenging it was, and I focused on how it was an amazing experience for me. I didn't need to do more. I did enough.

So for me, it wasn't about the summit. It was about the process of getting up there. And I think we can start to look at and appreciate our process in recovery as difficult as it may be, and it may be difficult for long periods of time.

And you may get to a point where you have to rest, where you have to stop, where you have to recalibrate. Where you might have to say, "I've gone far enough" in this particular area.

I was proud of stopping, I was proud that I didn't need to summit to be able to tell the stories to others, that I was able to take care of myself at that moment. At 65 I'm just not the young man I used to be. I don't need to take those risks to prove myself to others anymore. Recovery has taught me that, and in that moment I was grateful!

I had an enjoyable hike down the mountain. Going down was so relieving. And at no point did I shame myself or bad-mouth myself because I didn't summit.

In the past, summiting—getting to the top—was more about ego, showing off to others just for approval and to let people know that I did it.

Now I'm doing things for myself. And I'm learning to trust my own judgment about what's enough, what's too much, and what's just right.

There's a lesson in this for recovery. Sometimes perseverance means pushing through the hard parts. But sometimes it means knowing when to rest, when to regroup, when to try a different approach.

It's not about giving up. It's about being smart about how you use your energy. It's about playing the long game.

Because recovery isn't about one perfect day or one perfect decision. It's about thousands of imperfect days and millions of small decisions that, together, create a life worth living.

Reflection & Practice

Perseverance in recovery isn't about never falling. It's about getting back up when you fall.

Here are some questions to consider:

1. What's one area of your recovery where you've been tempted to give up?

2. What helps you stay the course when things get hard?

3. Think about a time you persevered through something difficult. What did you learn from that?

4. What's one small step you can take this week, even if it doesn't feel like enough?

Remember, recovery is cumulative. Every day you don't use, every honest conversation, every walk you take instead of giving in—that all stacks up.

Even on the days that feel small or useless, it matters.

You are not the same person you were yesterday.

You're building something.

Keep going.

Chapter Five:
Trust - Let the Process Work

Here's a truth a lot of people in recovery struggle with: you can't do this alone.

But—and this is just as important—not everyone gets to walk with you.

Trust is tricky. Especially when you've been hurt, let down, or abandoned. Especially when you've let yourself down. In early recovery, it's easy to swing too far in either direction: trusting no one... or trusting everyone.

The work is finding that middle ground.

I've seen both sides.

I've tried to muscle through recovery on my own. I've also tried to hand the wheel to people who had no business driving.

Neither one worked.

Real trust takes discernment. It means being open without being reckless. It means asking for help and keeping your eyes open. It means building relationships based on truth, not desperation.

"If I don't trust anyone, I stay isolated. If I trust too easily, I get used. Somewhere in between is where healing happens."

Letting Go of Control

In my adult life, I've often been fearful about running out. Running out of money, thinking will I be able to pay for this? Will I be able to pay for that? Will I have a job? Will I be able to make it?

I tried to force outcomes. And forcing outcomes is hard work.

I didn't necessarily get what I wanted when I was trying to force the situation. It was frustrating. It moved me away from spiritual principles because I wasn't always honest going about how I was getting what I wanted. I would leave things out. I probably rationalized and justified manipulative behavior. It led me to feel shame that I wasn't able to be consistent with my beliefs.

But when I realized—really realized—that there is a power greater than myself out there, everything changed. In early recovery, I intellectually recognized this, but later in recovery, it became deep. It became so deep that I no longer worried about money. I didn't have to force myself to get a 40-hour-a-week job and work for somebody else. I didn't have to wait to be discovered.

I trusted that the higher power, that energy, would provide for me.

Here's an example. One of my big complaints was that as a professional coach, I referred clients to different agencies—five, six, at a time. They would get their treatment there. But the agencies would never refer clients back to me.

I expected that this was a good deal for both ways and that they would reciprocate, but they didn't. I felt like it was unfair, or I was doing something wrong or was maybe not good enough to get the referrals back. Here I am putting all this energy into providing them with clients. But they wouldn't reciprocate.

And wow, I thought, how did I come to that conclusion after so many years of successfully working with clients.

Of course I was good enough. But I think what I was doing was relying on my will, my expectations and my small way of thinking to get business and the Universe wasn't paying me back exactly the way I thought it should. I was not trusting the process. My job is to put in the work but let go of the outcome. Because truth be told, regardless of those agencies not referring clients back to me, my schedule remained full. This reminds me of what someone told me a long time ago, "not to pray for what you want, because you don't know what's good for you." So, the idea is, to allow life and circumstances to happen as a result of the work you put in, and trust that all will be well in the end.

So when I started to trust the process, and let go and let GOD, I got what I needed. It didn't come from where I expected, it came from where it was supposed to come from. In recovery, they don't come in a straight line. They come from different places at different times, and in times when you wouldn't expect. But you can expect, that all will be well if you give time, time.

Also people would call me from 10, 15, even 20 years ago: "Michael, can I start seeing you again?" or "Michael, my aunt, my cousin needs some help. Can you talk to them?" The

Universe provides. So, my energy is better spent trusting that process instead of worrying about what I don't have.

It never ceases to amaze me how well I do when I'm focused on getting my work done, rather than consciously trying to make it happen. When I moved away from that idea—which for me was a lack of faith—good things started to happen.

Oh, and the idea that I had about being "discovered" that's never happened, not at least in the way you see in movies. I have always "been discovered," I just didn't realize it. I'm here, I'm seen, and the star that I am is enough.

Once again that old saying: "Faith moves mountains, but bring a shovel." While I'm still going to bring a shovel, I have faith that things are going to work out. I don't have to try and force outcomes to make them happen, but I still have to do the work!

Trust Without Guarantees

If you're going to trust recovery, you can't expect guarantees.

That's what makes it trust.

"The only way to trust, is to trust."

At my core, I know I can't predict or control the future. I don't know what my life will look like at 80. I don't know if I'll be physically fit and able. I don't know if I'll have money. I don't know any of that.

But the very best I can do now is work on my physical fitness, develop myself spiritually, mentally, emotionally, and financially today because that's all I have. I do my best to eat well. I meditate regularly. I journal regularly. I talk honestly to people, and I try to clear a way for a better tomorrow.

I put energy into revealing myself to people where in the past I kept many secrets. When I'm holding things in, I'm not free. When I let them go, I've got energy and lightness, and I can move on.

I try my best to be an open book and be honest and authentic. And the truth is, I couldn't do that 10 years ago. I wasn't able to do that 20 years ago. But I'm doing it now. And the now is what's real.

Trust is about being vulnerable even when it's uncomfortable. It's about putting yourself out there even when there are no guarantees. It's about showing up authentically, even when it seems easier to hide.

"The hardest part of recovery wasn't trusting other people. It was learning to trust myself"

When Help Comes From Unexpected Places

I have a story I like to tell about trust in recovery that might surprise you.

Early in my recovery, I ended up in a therapeutic community. I walked in thinking I didn't belong. I wasn't like "those people." They had criminal backgrounds, they were poor, they were uneducated. At least from my prejudgment. I mean how the hell did I know where all these people came from and what their backgrounds were. Sometimes my prejudgment seems to only provide me comfort for that moment but is so distorted and untrue.

And rather than identify with my peers at that rehab, I wanted to maintain my uniqueness, indifference. I was convinced that I was better than them, somehow in some way very, very special.

But over time, all that seemed to change because the truth was, I was like them more than not. When I was able to connect on a feelings level, I saw how I could be helped, and I was able to help.

They taught me more than any textbook ever could. They showed me what honesty looks like. That showing vulnerability was a practice of courage and not of weakness.

That's when I started to understand trust.

Not blind trust. But earned trust.

And that's a big part of what I do in my work now. I talk a lot about involving the whole family in the recovery journey, not just the person struggling.

Why? Because trust has usually been broken on all sides. And healing that hurt takes more than one person.

Everyone has a role. Everyone needs support. Everyone needs a space to be honest.

Trust doesn't mean pretending everything's fine.

It means telling the truth, consistently, until it becomes the new normal.

I've had a total knee replacement. I've had cancer. I have thyroid problems. I have vision problems. But every opportunity to get help for these issues has been provided for me.

I haven't had to struggle or force things to happen. I've just had to be available for what I call the miracle. I've just walked through the door. That door will be there; just go through it.

Even as I talk about this, I feel so much gratitude. I wonder sometimes how I'm so fortunate. I'm not some big shot, wealthy millionaire, billionaire, or famous person. I'm just a regular guy who lives a great life. How have I been afforded this great life?

I believe there is a power greater than myself that's helping me along. But 50% of it is me. I'm doing some work for this to happen too. As long as I do my part, I'm going to be okay, and faith and trust will take care of the rest.

You have to put some effort into this. It's not going to happen just because you want it to. The other thing I've come to understand is the idea of prayer—what do I know? I don't know for what to pray for. If you leave it up to me, I'm going to pray for all the wrong things.

I pray that light shines over me and moves me in the direction I need to go, and gives me exactly what I need.

Working With (Not Against) Your Higher Power

Self-trust gets rebuilt the same way trust between people does: through consistent action.

Keep your word. Say what you mean. Follow through. Own your mistakes. Celebrate your wins. Pay attention to what your body is telling you.

You don't have to be perfect. Just honest. Just willing.

Some people will leave your life when you get into recovery. That's okay.

Some relationships were only possible because of the version of you that was still numbing, still performing, still afraid.

Let them go.

Other people will surprise you. They'll show up. They'll hold you accountable. They'll root for you in quiet ways you never expected.

Let them in.

This path wasn't meant to be walked alone.

Just walk it with people who are walking it too.

And don't be too quick to dismiss the signs that show up in your life. The people who appear at just the right moment. The opportunities that come out of nowhere. The doors that open when others close.

These aren't coincidences. They're evidence of something working in your life that's bigger than you.

Call it God, the Universe, a higher power, energy, light, love— whatever works for you.

The name doesn't matter. What matters is recognizing that you're not alone in this.

There is help available. There is hope available. There is healing available.

But you have to be willing to receive it. You have to be willing to trust it. You have to be willing to work with it, not against it.

When I look back at my recovery journey, I can see so clearly the moments when I was fighting the current: trying to force things, manipulate outcomes, control what wasn't mine to control.

And I can see just as clearly the moments when I surrendered to the flow—when I trusted the process, when I did the right thing, and allowed life to unfold.

The difference is night and day.

In those moments of surrender and trust, life opened up in ways I never could have orchestrated on my own. Doors opened. People appeared. Resources materialized. Not because I was special or deserving, but because that's how life works when we get out of our own way.

Trust doesn't mean passivity. It doesn't mean sitting back and waiting for someone or something to save you. It means doing your part and trusting that the Universe will meet you halfway. It means showing up fully and letting go of the outcome. It means working hard and surrendering the results.

It's a delicate balance, this dance between effort and surrender. But it's where the magic happens. It's where recovery becomes not just a struggle to stay clean, but a journey of discovery, growth, and transformation.

Reflection & Practice

Trust in recovery is a practice, not a destination. It's something you build over time, through consistent action and reflection.

Here are some questions to consider:

1. Who do you truly trust right now, and why?

2. Where have you ignored your instincts in the past, and what did that teach you?

3. What would it look like to take one step toward building trust with someone in your life?

4. What's one thing you can do this week to build self-trust?

Trust is the foundation of any meaningful relationship, including the one you have with yourself. It's not about being perfect or never making mistakes. It's about being honest, showing up, and doing your best.

Start small. Trust yourself to keep one promise today. Trust someone else with one small truth. See what opens up when you do.

You're not alone. But you do get to choose who walks with you.

Chapter Six:
Humility – The Strength to Learn from Everyone

I used to think humility meant weakness.

That it meant shrinking, lowering your head, letting other people talk over you. But I've learned that humility is actually a kind of strength—a quiet confidence in knowing you don't have all the answers, but also knowing you have some of them.

In recovery, humility isn't optional. It's foundational.

Because without it, you won't take suggestions. You won't hear feedback. You won't ask for help. And you'll miss out on the very relationships and experiences that could save your life.

"When I think I know everything, I stop learning. When I stop learning, I stop growing."

When I was new in recovery, I didn't want to be told what to do. I didn't want to admit I was struggling. I didn't want to sit in a room full of people I thought were beneath me.

And I definitely didn't want to hear advice from someone who didn't have the same background, education, or life experience as me.

But here's the truth: some of the wisest things I've ever heard came from people who weren't like me: some rich, some poor, some old, some young, some Indian, some Asian, some that were highly educated, and some that didn't finish high school.

People who spoke with more heart than polish.

Their honesty cracked something open in me.

Because when someone tells the truth—without ego, without performance—you feel it. And it gives you permission to do the same.

So sometimes I just shut my eyes and listened. That way it's easier to hear the message.

Humility isn't just theoretical in my life. It shows up in concrete, sometimes uncomfortable ways.

As I talked about earlier when I shared my experience of climbing Mount Meru; and by the way, I had a similar experience climbing Machu Picchu, but we won't talk about that now.

It's not about thinking less of yourself. It's about thinking of yourself accurately. It's about seeing yourself clearly—strengths and weaknesses, gifts and limitations—and working with what you have, not what you wish you had.

And there's freedom in that. When I stopped trying to be the strongest, the fastest, the best, I could just be me. I could enjoy the journey, appreciate the experience, and find joy in the process, even when it was hard. Even when I was last.

That's the paradox of humility: when you accept your limitations, you actually become stronger. You become more resilient. You become more capable of growth and change.

Because you're no longer wasting energy pretending to be something you're not.

The Gift of Being Wrong

One of the practices I come back to again and again is asking myself: What don't I know yet?

That question keeps me grounded. It keeps me open. It reminds me that every person I meet, every challenge I face, every mistake I make... has something to teach me.

Humility isn't about playing small. It's about staying open.

I've worked with CEOs and clinicians, teachers and truck drivers, parents and parolees—and here's what I know:

Everyone is trying to figure something out.

No one has it all together.

And the minute you think you're above learning from someone else, you close the door on your own growth.

"You can learn something from anyone—if you're willing to listen."

I remember when I first started working as a therapist in New York. I was 34 years old, Black, working in an agency that was probably 85% white. And I got this client who owned a bank. This guy owns a bank, and I'm his therapist.

There was a part of me that thought, "He should be telling me what to do. How am I guiding this person that owns a bank?"

I had clients who were lawyers, doctors, and famous people I'd seen on TV. I had people that represented my grandfather, grandmother, mother, and father. All of these people that were, on some level in life, "superior" to me were now listening to me.

I had to make an adjustment. I had to rise up and not look up to people. I had to level myself and see people as equals. I wasn't better than them, and they weren't better than me. I had a job to do, and I had to take on the role of their guide. I didn't know a lot about banking, but I did know about the recovery process and that's how I could help them. So, the things that I didn't know weren't applicable to this situation. What I did know was exactly what was needed.

That was one of my first examples of humility. For me, humility wasn't about lowering myself. It was about raising myself up and acknowledging my strength which then made me equal to the person I was there to help.

This is the work of humility in recovery. It's about finding that middle ground where you're not above anyone, but you're not below anyone either. You're just human, like everyone else. Equal in dignity, equal in value, equal in worth.

And from that place of equality, you can both give and receive. You can help others, and you can let others help you. You can teach, and you can learn. You can speak, and you can listen.

That's where the real connection happens. That's where the real work is. That's where recovery truly begins.

Learning from Those You Least Expect

Recovery is one big humility practice.

It asks you to be honest about your past, flexible in your present, and curious about your future.

You'll mess up. You'll circle back. You'll think you've got it down... and then life will show you another layer to work on.

That's not failure. That's being human. That's how life works.

I mentioned earlier that when I was first sent to a therapeutic community, I walked in thinking I didn't belong there. I was convinced that I was different.

But that was just my ego talking. That was my fear. That was my unwillingness to look at myself.

Because the truth was, I did belong there. I needed exactly what that place had to offer—structure, accountability, community, and a mirror that wouldn't let me hide from myself.

Those men and women, whom I initially judged as beneath me, became some of my greatest teachers. They showed me what raw honesty looks like. They showed me what accountability means. They showed me that recovery isn't about being perfect; it's about being real.

I had to let go of my preconceptions. I had to let go of my judgments. I had to let go of the story I was telling myself about who I was and who I thought they were.

And when I did, I found a connection. I found understanding. I found a shared humanity that transcended our differences.

That's the gift of humility. It opens you up to learning from everyone, especially from those you least expect to learn from.

So, who are you dismissing right now? Who are you judging as not worth listening to? Who are you writing off as too different, too difficult, too damaged to teach you anything?

That person might be holding exactly the insight you need to hear.

But you'll never know unless you're humble enough to listen.

Why Vulnerability Isn't Weakness

There's also a kind of humility in joy.

In letting yourself be seen. In receiving compliments. In celebrating a win without brushing it off or explaining it away.

"I used to think I didn't deserve praise. Now I try to take it in. That's humility, too."

This may seem counterintuitive. How is accepting praise an act of humility?

Because it acknowledges that we don't get to decide how others see us. It acknowledges that we're not the final authority on our own worth. It acknowledges that sometimes, others see gifts in us that we can't see in ourselves.

I remember talking with Matt Williams on his podcast. He introduced me as a special guest, and right away, I acknowledged that when he used the word "special," it hit me in a certain way.

I was raised to believe that since you're supposed to do the right thing, you don't get credit for doing it because you're supposed to do it anyway. And so, I haven't really been able to experience the acknowledgment that people have given me for the positive things I've done, I haven't been able to really experience it.

"Wow, that really feels good to know that somebody thinks I'm special."

So, there's been a big part of my life that I've missed—the goodness that other people offer me was a truth that I denied. The truth of my greatness or that part of me that's special.

I'm now starting to truly acknowledge when somebody says something complimentary, and really take it in rather than just blowing it off. Sometimes I would tell myself they're just saying that because that's what they're supposed to say, but now I'm really starting to take it in.

This is part of humility too—allowing others to see us, to know us, to celebrate us. Not because we need their approval, but because connection is a two-way street. It requires not just giving, but receiving as well.

In my work with clients, I often see this struggle. People in recovery want to help others, want to make amends, want to give back. But they struggle to receive help, to accept forgiveness, to take in appreciation.

They think humility means always serving, never being served. Always giving, never receiving. Always lifting others up, never being lifted up themselves.

But that's not humility. That's just another form of control. That's just another way of keeping walls up, of staying safe, of avoiding vulnerability.

True humility means allowing yourself to be seen—fully, authentically, with all your strengths and all your weaknesses. It means letting yourself be human in front of other humans.

There's strength in that. There's courage in that. There's recovery in that.

Reflection & Practice

Humility in recovery isn't about making yourself small. It's about making room for growth, for connection, for transformation.

Here are some questions to consider:

1. Where in your life have you confused humility with weakness?

2. Who has taught you something meaningful, even if they weren't someone you'd expected to learn from?

3. What's one area where you could practice more curiosity instead of control?

4. What truth about yourself are you ready to acknowledge and own?

Humility isn't something you achieve once and for all. It's a daily practice, a moment-by-moment choice to stay open, stay honest, stay willing to learn and grow.

Start small. Notice when your ego flares up. Notice when you're tempted to dismiss someone or something. Notice when you feel the need to prove yourself or defend yourself or make yourself feel either bigger or smaller than you actually are.

And in those moments, take a breath. Step back. Ask yourself: What's the humble response here? What's the response that makes space for growth, for connection, for truth?

That's where recovery lives. That's where healing happens. That's where transformation begins.

Stay open. Stay teachable. Stay honest.

That's humility.

Chapter Seven:
The Three Phases of Recovery

Recovery isn't a single event—it's a journey with distinct phases. Understanding where you are in that journey can help you find the right tools, set realistic expectations, and keep moving forward when the path gets hard.

In my work with clients—and in my own experience—I've noticed three main phases that most people go through: Recognizing the Problem, Getting Unstuck and Taking Action, and Keep Moving Forward. This can be at any stage of your recovery depending on what you're working on.

Each phase has its own challenges, its own opportunities, and its own tools for success. And while not everyone's journey looks exactly the same, recognizing these patterns can help you navigate your own path with more clarity and confidence.

Let's explore each phase together, and then talk about how to create a recovery plan that actually works for where you are right now.

Phase One: Recognizing the Problem (Abstinence & Discovery)

The foundation of recovery is stopping the behavior and starting the self-discovery.

Abstinence is what gives you clarity. Without it, you can't really see what's happening. But abstinence alone isn't enough. Once you stop the behavior, the real work begins.

Discovery is the process of asking, Who am I underneath the patterns? It's how you start building a life that's worth living.

When I was first getting clean, I wasn't thinking about the rest of my life. I was thinking about today. Just today. Can I make it through today without using? That was enough of a challenge.

For most people who are just getting into recovery, that's where you need to start. Simple abstinence. A clear commitment to stop and stay stopped—one day at a time.

But alongside that commitment, you need to start the process of discovery. Who are you without the substance? What triggers your desire to use? What helps you stay clean?

In this phase, it's helpful to:

• Identify your patterns—what are you using to numb or avoid? What are the people, places and things that trigger you.

• Make a clear commitment to stop, one day at a time, an hour at a time, a minute at a time, or a second at a time.

• Replace the habit with reflection: journaling, walking, talking, listening, being quiet.

• Pay attention to what you feel, not just what you do.

This isn't about being "good." It's about being honest.

When people ask me how long this phase lasts, I usually say about nine months. That's just a guideline, not a rule. Some people move through it faster; some people stay here longer.

The key is to remember that these first nine months aren't recovery—they're discovery. You're just starting to figure things out. You're just starting to build a foundation. You're just starting to understand what recovery might look like for you.

Be patient with yourself. Be honest with yourself. And be willing to try things, even things that don't immediately make sense or feel comfortable.

This is where you start to break the isolation, reach out for help, and build a support system that works for you. This is where you start to learn new coping skills, new ways of thinking, new ways of being in the world.

It's messy. It's confusing. Sometimes it's incredibly painful.

But it's also where the magic begins.

Phase Two: Getting Unstuck and Taking Action

Once you've been in recovery for a while—you have some clean time, you've started to build a support system, you've begun to understand your patterns—you might find yourself hitting a plateau.

The initial urgency of getting clean has passed. The daily struggle has become more manageable. But now you're facing a different challenge: you're stuck.

Maybe you're stuck in old patterns of thinking, even though your behavior has changed. Maybe you're stuck in unhealthy relationships that no longer serve you. Maybe you're stuck in a job that drains you, a living situation that stresses you, or a routine that's become more about survival than growth.

This is the Getting Unstuck phase.

It's where you go deeper. It's where you start to address not just the behavior, but the underlying issues that drove the behavior in the first place. It's where you start to build not just a clean life, but a meaningful one.

For me, this phase was about asking tough questions: What am I still holding onto that doesn't serve me? What am I afraid to let go of? What am I afraid to try? What am I avoiding?

It was also about taking risks—creative risks, emotional risks, social risks. It was about pushing beyond my comfort zone and exploring new parts of myself.

In this phase, it helps to:

• Identify what's keeping you stuck—What old patterns, beliefs, or relationships are holding you back?

• Take new risks—What have you always wanted to try but been afraid to?

• Deepen your work—Therapy, journaling, meditation, service work, therapeutic retreats—whatever helps you continue to grow.

• Build healthier relationships—With yourself, with others, with a higher power.

This is often where people start to discover their passions, their purpose, their unique gifts. It's where recovery becomes not just about staying clean, but about building a life that's worth living.

For me, it was in this phase that I started to pursue adventure in a serious way. I discovered my love for hiking, for travel, for pushing my physical limits. I started to see myself as an athlete, an explorer, a person capable of more than I'd ever imagined.

It was also in this phase that I deepened my spiritual practice. I learned to meditate, to journal more consistently, to connect with a higher power in a way that felt authentic and meaningful to me. I also developed and practiced manifestation.

And it was in this phase that I started to rebuild relationships—not just with others, but with myself. I learned to speak to myself with more kindness, to trust my own judgment, to honor my own needs and boundaries.

The Getting Unstuck phase is where recovery starts to become truly yours. Not something you're doing because someone else told you to, but something you're building because you want to.

Phase Three: Keep Moving Forward

The third phase of recovery is about sustainability, perseverance, and continued growth. It's about building a life that supports your recovery for the long haul.

This is where you are after you've done a lot of the hard work. You've gotten clean. You've built a support system. You've addressed underlying issues. You've started to discover who you are without the substance.

Now the question becomes: How do you keep it moving? How do you sustain this recovery for years, decades, a lifetime, a day at a time?

The Keep Moving Forward phase is about:

• Building routines that support your recovery—Not rigid rules, but rhythms that help you stay grounded.

• Continuing to grow and evolve—Trying new things, learning new skills, exploring new parts of yourself.

• Giving back—Sharing your experience, strength, and hope with others.

• Finding balance—Between work and rest, solitude and connection, giving and receiving.

"A good deal, is a good deal, for both" - Robert Smith

For me, this phase has been about finding ways to challenge myself without burning myself out. It's been about building a life that's full and meaningful, but also sustainable.

I run ultra-marathons, but I also make sure I get enough rest. I travel to remote places, but I also maintain connections at home. I give to others, but I also make sure my own cup is full.

It's a balancing act, and I don't always get it right. There are still days when I feel stuck, days when I struggle, days when I wonder if I'm on the right path.

But the difference is that now I have tools. I have support. I have experience. I know what works for me, and I know what doesn't. I know how to course-correct when I get off track.

And most importantly, I know that recovery isn't a destination—it's an ongoing journey of growth, discovery, and transformation.

Creating Your Own Recovery Plan

Now that you understand the three phases of recovery, let's talk about how to create a plan that works for where you are right now.

First, it's important to be honest about which phase you're in. Are you just getting started? Are you stuck in old patterns despite having some clean time? Are you working on sustainability and long-term growth?

Wherever you are, that's okay. There's no right or wrong place to be. What matters is that you're willing to start from where you are.

Once you've identified your phase, you can start to build a plan that addresses your specific needs.

If you're in Phase One (Recognizing the Problem), your plan might focus on:

• Building a daily routine that supports abstinence.

• Finding a support system—whether that's a 12-step group, a therapy group, or a few trusted friends.

• Learning basic coping skills for managing cravings and triggers. Whether it be food, money, sex, internet, or control.

• Starting to explore who you are without the substance, without the behavior.

If you're in Phase Two (Getting Unstuck and Taking Action) your plan might focus on:

• Deepening your self-awareness through therapy, journaling, or meditation.

• Taking creative risks and exploring new interests.

• Addressing underlying trauma or emotional issues.

• Building healthier relationships and setting better boundaries.

If you're in Phase Three (Keep Moving Forward), your plan might focus on:

• Refining your daily practices to support long-term sustainability.

• Finding ways to give back and share your experience with others.

• Continuing to grow and evolve in all areas of your life.

• Building a life that's meaningful and fulfilling, beyond just staying clean.

Remember, this plan isn't set in stone. It's a living document that will evolve as you do. The key is to start somewhere and be willing to adjust as you go.

It's also important to remember that recovery isn't linear. You might move back and forth between phases. You might have days where you feel like you're starting over. That's okay.

Recovery is messy. It's not about doing it perfectly—it's about doing it consistently, with honesty and courage.

And it's about finding what works for you. Not what worked for someone else, unless of course that works for you. Understand your unique challenges, your unique strengths. Your journey is yours.

Because your recovery is your responsibility, and no one else's.

Reflection & Practice

Take some time to reflect on where you are in your recovery journey:

1. Which phase do you think you're in right now— Recognizing the Problem, Getting Unstuck and Taking Action, or Keep Moving Forward? What makes you say that?

2. What's working well for you in this phase? What's challenging?

3. What's one small step you could take this week to support your growth in this phase?

4. Who can help you in this phase? Who might be able to offer guidance, support, or accountability?

Now, start to sketch out a simple recovery plan for yourself. It doesn't have to be elaborate or perfect. Just a basic outline of:

• Your daily practices (what will you do each day to support your recovery?)

• Your weekly practices (what will you do each week to deepen your recovery?)

• Your emergency plan (what will you do when things get hard?)

• Your support team (who can you reach out to when you need help?)

Remember, this plan isn't about restricting yourself or boxing yourself in. It's about creating a structure that supports your freedom and growth.

It's about building a life that's worth staying clean for.

What will that look like for you?

Chapter Eight:
When You Fall Off
(And How to Get Back Up)

L et's get something straight right now: slipping doesn't mean it's over.

There's this belief, especially early on, that if you mess up, if you relapse, if you break your commitment, you've ruined everything. You haven't.

Recovery isn't about never falling. It's about learning how to get back up.

"What matters most isn't the mistake—it's what you do next."

Everyone drifts. Everyone has days or weeks when they go quiet, pull away, or slip back into old habits.

The key is to notice it, name it, and course-correct before you spiral out of control.

This chapter is about how to do that.

The Reality of Setbacks

First, let's talk about what a setback actually is. Because it's not just about returning to substance use, though that's certainly one form.

A setback can be:

• Using again after a period of abstinence

• Falling back into old thought patterns or behaviors

• Isolating yourself from support

• Stopping the practices that have been helping you

• Lying to yourself or others about how you're doing

All of these are signs that you're drifting off course. And all of them are normal, human responses to stress, fear, or pain.

The problem isn't that setbacks happen. The problem is what we make them mean.

If you see a setback as proof that you're a failure, that recovery is impossible, that you might as well give up, then a small slip can quickly become a full-blown relapse.

But if you see a setback as information—as data about what's not working, what triggers you, what you need to address—then it can actually strengthen your recovery in the long run.

I've seen people who've been clean for years suddenly slip. And I've seen how differently that can play out.

Some people spiral into shame, hide from their support system, and end up in a worse place than where they started. They allow fear to take over. So the question is, "Can you be afraid, and do the work anyway?" - Vincent Casaloro

Others acknowledge what happened, reach out for help, learn from the experience, and come back stronger than before.

The difference isn't in the slip itself. It's in the response.

Why "Forever" Thinking Doesn't Help

One of the things that makes slips so devastating is the way we talk about recovery—as this all-or-nothing, perfect-or-failed proposition.

"I have to stay clean forever." "I can never use again." "One slip and I'm back to zero."

This kind of thinking sets us up for failure. Because forever is a long time. And never is a heavy word.

When I work with clients, I encourage them to focus on today. Just today. Can you stay clean today? Can you make good choices today? Can you reach out for help today?

That's not to say long-term recovery isn't the goal. It absolutely is. But you don't get there by fixating on forever. You get there by stringing together a series of todays.

I think one of the things that scares people about recovery is the term "long term." People don't want to get into this thing for the rest of their life. Or at least, I didn't. I wanted the pain to stop. I certainly wasn't thinking, "Oh, I want to stop for the rest of my life, and I want to stop everything."

I think when you throw that in someone's face, it turns them off.

What was helpful for me wasn't so much the "one day at a time" mantra—that seemed pretty silly at first. It was knowing that my life would improve if I stopped. It was seeing the concrete benefits, the payoff, of staying clean.

So, if you're struggling, don't think about forever. Think about today. Think about what you gain by staying clean today. Think about what you lose by going back today.

"Play the tape, all the way through." - Anonymous

And remember that nobody, not even people with decades of recovery, has figured out how to do this perfectly. We're all just trying to make the next right choice, a day at a time.

The Five Steps to Course Correction

When you do slip—and at some point, in some way, most of us do—there's a process you can follow to get back on track. I call it course correction, and it works whether you've fully relapsed or just notice yourself drifting toward old patterns.

Step 1: Name What's Happening

If you've returned to using—or just checked out emotionally— don't sugarcoat it. Don't justify it. And don't wait too long to say it out loud.

Say it to yourself first: "I slipped. I messed up."

Then say it to someone you trust.

Shame feeds on secrecy. The moment you name it, you take away its power.

This is the hardest step for most people because it requires vulnerability. It requires admitting that you're not perfect, that you're struggling, that you need help.

But it's also the most powerful step. Because once you name what's happening, you can start to address it. You may not understand it at first, but you can start to change it.

Step 2: Pause the Panic

You don't need to make twelve huge changes overnight. You just need to stop the bleeding.

• Get back to basics: food, water, sleep, connection

• Reach out to a human being—even if it's just to say, "I'm not okay"

• Stay away from people, places and things that keep you stuck

This is triage. Stabilize first.

When we're in crisis, our tendency is to either overreact or underreact. We either try to change everything at once—which isn't sustainable—or we convince ourselves it's not that bad and keep going down the same path.

Neither approach works.

Instead, focus on the essentials. What do you need right now to stabilize? What are one or two things you can do today to stop things from getting worse?

Maybe it's calling for support. Maybe it's calling a sponsor. Maybe it's going to a meeting. Maybe it's going to detox. Or maybe it's just as simple as getting a good night's sleep so you can think more clearly. You put together what works for you.

Whatever it is, do that first. Then you can start to address the bigger issues.

Step 3: Reflect—Without Self-Destruction

Once the dust settles, ask yourself:

• What led up to this?

• What was I feeling that I didn't want to feel?

• What did I stop doing that had been helping me?

This isn't about punishment—it's about information.

Every setback holds a clue about what you need.

This is where a lot of people get stuck. They either skip reflection altogether, afraid to look too closely at what happened, or they use reflection as a weapon against themselves, beating themselves up for every mistake and weakness.

Neither approach helps.

Effective reflection is curious, not judgmental. It asks, "What happened here? What can I learn from this?" not "What's wrong with me? Why can't I get this right?"

It's about understanding patterns, triggers, and needs—not assigning blame or shame.

Step 4: Recommit

Recommitment isn't a grand speech or a perfect plan. It's a decision:

"I'm getting back on the path—starting today."

What helps:

• Return to your three-part plan from the last chapter

• Call your coach or therapist, make a meeting, call a support

• Reset your space: clean up, write down your thoughts or feelings, breathe

It doesn't have to be dramatic. It just has to be real.

Recommitment is about action, not words. It's about doing something—even something small—that puts you back on the path of recovery.

Maybe it's going to a meeting. Maybe it's calling your sponsor. Maybe it's journaling about what you want for your life. Maybe it's just getting back to the daily practices that have helped you stay clean in the past.

The action itself matters less than the intention behind it: I am choosing recovery, again, today.

Step 5: Build Back Stronger

This is where you take what you've learned and reinforce your foundation.

• Do you need more structure?

- A different support group?

- A better nighttime routine?

- To finally tell the truth about something?

You don't go back to square one. You go back wiser.

"Slipping doesn't erase your progress. It refines your approach."

This is the step that transforms a setback from a failure into an opportunity for growth. It's where you use what you've learned to strengthen your recovery, to build a foundation that can withstand similar challenges in the future.

Maybe you realize you need more support on weekends. Maybe you need better boundaries with certain people. Maybe you need to address an underlying issue in therapy. Maybe you need to find a physical outlet for stress. Maybe the answer is to return to a treatment program that specifically addresses your issues, not just a general disease concept model. If you have issues with trauma, mental health, and family and they go unaddressed a return to using can happen.

Have you ever thought about planning your next relapse? And what do the people around you need to do in response once they find out? Would they call your sponsor? Would they come to your house and give you support? Would they take you to a place where you feel safe? And if you put that together guess what? You won't have to do it alone.

Whatever it is, this is your chance to build a recovery that's not just about not using, but about truly thriving.

Building a Better Support System

One of the most important factors in how well you recover from a setback is the quality of your support system. Not just how many people you have around you, but who they are and how they show up for you.

A good support system doesn't shame you when you slip. They don't say, "I knew you couldn't do it" or "You've really messed up this time." They say, "I'm glad you told me. What do you need? How can I help? What's next?"

They hold you accountable without making you feel worthless. They believe in your capacity to recover, even when you don't believe in yourself. They see the slip as a moment, not a definition.

If your current support system isn't helping you get back up when you fall, it might be time to make some changes. That doesn't necessarily mean cutting people off, but it might mean expanding your circle to include others who understand you and your recovery needs better.

This could mean finding a new meeting, a new therapist, a new sponsor. It could mean finding a group therapy that can support your recovery or new friends who are on a similar path. It could mean being more selective about who you share your struggles with, focusing on people who respond with compassion and wisdom rather than judgment or enabling.

Remember, it's okay to curate your support system. It's okay to set boundaries with people who aren't helpful. It's okay to seek out those who have what you want—stability, peace, joy, connection—and ask them to help you find your way there too.

Your recovery depends on it.

If You're Reading This After a Setback

If you're reading this chapter after experiencing a setback—whether it was five minutes ago or five years ago—I want you to hear this:

You're not broken. You're not a failure. You're human.

Come back. You're still in this.

Recovery is not about being flawless. It's about trusting a process that can work and help you grow.

You're not starting over. You're starting again—with more clarity than before.

What if I Did Know?

During my time living in New York City and going through my first five years of recovery, I learned something really important from Milton Smith, LCSW, a therapist who helped me in those early days. Whenever I answered his questions with "I don't know," he would challenge me with, "Well, what if you did know?" This question had a huge impact on me. It pushed me to stop being lazy and start thinking actively about solutions.

This idea of "What if you did know?" is like a spark that encourages me to think deeper and explore new possibilities. When I'm faced with uncertainty, instead of getting stuck, I can imagine different scenarios and draw on my intuition. It's a way to shift from feeling limited to realizing there's potential for discovery. This approach is especially useful when I need to solve problems or think creatively.

When I started to think about what I might know, it opened up a whole new world of ideas and insights that I hadn't considered before. It turned conversations from feeling like dead ends into pathways for discovery. I learned that instead of just accepting that I didn't have the answers, I could explore my experiences and beliefs to find new solutions.

In a group setting, this technique really helped me when I was feeling overwhelmed. Instead of freezing up because of what I said I didn't know, I could reflect on the possibility of what I might know and how it could apply in different situations. This approach created some really deep, insightful, and emotional therapy group sessions where curiosity thrives, and everyone feels encouraged to share their thoughts. During group, asking "What if you did know?" can be a game-changer. It can get everyone brainstorming together, combining our different ideas to come up with solutions. This way, it feels less like an individual struggle and more like a team effort, where we all contribute to finding answers.

On a personal level, this mindset has helped me deal with self-doubt and insecurity. Instead of feeling stuck by my uncertainties, I can challenge myself to think about my potential and my goals. This shift in thinking opens up a path for personal growth and self-discovery.

Philosophically, this question makes me think about knowledge itself. It invites me to consider that what I think I know might just be the starting point for more exploration. This kind of reflection has led to discussions about how recovery works and what it is that I need to do to improve, along with understanding me better.

In creative pursuits, this approach can be a powerful tool. Whether I'm journaling, meditating, engaged in an art project, gardening, or figuring out how I can be helpful in a situation, asking "What if you did know?" helps me break through blocks and tap into my creativity. It encourages me to trust my instincts and see the unknown as a source of inspiration.

Overall, the invitation to think about what I might know in the face of uncertainty builds resilience and adaptability. It teaches me to see challenges as opportunities for growth and exploration. Whether in personal development, educational courses, teamwork, or creative projects, this simple yet profound question transforms how I engage with knowledge and possibility, unlocking the potential that lies within uncertainty.

Reflection & Practice

Take some time to reflect on your own experience with setbacks:

1. Think about a time when you've slipped or relapsed in the past. What did you learn from that experience?

2. What are your early warning signs that you might be headed toward a setback? How can you catch them sooner?

3. Who are the people in your life who help you get back up when you fall? How can you strengthen those

connections?

4. If you struggle with any of the above questions, ask yourself, "What if you did know?"

Now, create a simple "emergency plan" for yourself—a list of actions you can take if you feel yourself slipping. This might include:

• People to call

• Meetings to attend

• Tools to use

• Places to go (or avoid)

• Reminders of why recovery matters to you

Keep this plan somewhere accessible—on your phone, in your wallet, in your glove compartment, anywhere so you can turn to it when you need it most.

Remember, setbacks don't define you. Your response to them does.

And with the right tools, the right support, and the right attitude, you can turn any setback into a stepping stone toward a stronger recovery.

Chapter Nine:
The Family is The Addict, The Addict is The Family, We're All in This Together

Recovery doesn't happen in isolation. Neither does addiction, although at the core of addiction is often loneliness, a close relative of isolation.

When someone is caught in addiction, everyone around them is affected. Parents, children, partners, siblings, friends, co-workers, and even strangers—they all experience the ripple effects. They develop their own coping mechanisms, their own ways of responding to the chaos, their own wounds that need healing.

Let's face it, as a family member addiction has negatively affected your life, and often choosing to help the addict or the alcoholic, and not getting help for yourself. Everyone needs the opportunity to recover.

I learned this both from my own experience and from working with hundreds of families over the years. Time and again, I've seen how addiction becomes a family disease and how recovery must be a family process.

How Addiction Affects Everyone

Let me paint a picture for you.

Joe is a husband and father who's been struggling with alcohol for years. It started with a few drinks after work to "take the edge off." Then it was a six-pack every night or most nights. Then it was missing work or deadlines at work, hiding bottles, and lying about where he's been.

His wife, Sarah, starts covering for him. She makes excuses when he misses family events. She takes on extra work when he inevitably loses his job. The fighting starts and she's walking on eggshells to avoid triggering his anger. She's exhausted, resentful, and scared—but she tells herself she's just being supportive. She may also just keep quiet. If he's the breadwinner and she doesn't want to piss him off.

Their teenage daughter, Emma, becomes the perfect student. Straight A's, never causes trouble, takes care of her younger brother. She thinks if she's good enough, maybe her dad will stop drinking. Or at the very least, her mom will notice her. At night, she lies awake listening to them arguing and fighting.

Their son, Tyler, goes the opposite direction. He acts out at school, gets in fights, starts experimenting with drugs himself. It's his way of screaming, "Something is wrong in our family! Someone please notice!"

Sarah's parents get involved. They lend money, offer advice. They judge Joe harshly while enabling the situation to continue. They think they're helping, but they're really just getting pulled into the problem.

This isn't just Joe's problem. It's the family's problem. And every person in this scenario needs help.

The family members of an addict or alcoholic often experience the same emotional, psychological, and physical symptoms as the addict himself. The addict has poor boundaries; the family has poor boundaries. The addict engages in denial; the family engages in denial. The addict isolates; the family isolates. Here is a list of consequences the family goes through, see if you've experienced any:

- Increased stress

- Problems sleeping

- Fatigue

- Headaches

- Gastrointestinal issues

- Weakened immune system

- Chronic pain

- Weight changes

- Substance use

- Cardiovascular issues

- Anxiety

- Depression

- Guilt and shame

- Low self-esteem

- Fear

- Anger and resentments

- Post-Traumatic stress

- Difficulty trusting others

- Not living within your value system

Everyone is responding to the crisis in the family in negative ways and is paying the price for untreated addiction.

I often see family members eating too much or too little, struggling to sleep, having difficulty concentrating, experiencing financial problems, isolating from friends, showing mood swings, or acting out with inappropriate behaviors. Sound familiar? Those are the same symptoms we see in addiction.

That's why we say the family is the addict. Because everyone has been affected. And everyone needs to heal.

Breaking the Enablement Cycle

One of the most difficult patterns to break in families affected by addiction is enabling. Enabling happens when, in an effort to help, we actually make it easier for the addicted person to continue using. We remove consequences. We solve problems. We make excuses. We clean up messes—literally and figuratively. We do for the addict what they can most likely do for themselves.

We think we're helping. We're not.

I've worked with family members who pay the rent, the car note, the phone bill for their addicted loved one who's in rehab. They're still being affected by the addiction. "I have to pay the rent while they're in rehab," they think. "I have to make sure they have a place to go when they get out."

But when do they start to recover from feeling responsible for somebody else? When do they get to focus on their own well-being?

I remember working with a mother who was sending money to her addicted son. She was on a fixed income, barely making ends meet, but still sending hundreds of dollars a month to her 35-year-old son who was actively using.

"I can't let him be homeless," she told me.

"Is he homeless now?" I asked.

"No, he lives with his girlfriend."

"So, what's the money for?"

"Well, he says it's for food and bills, but..." she trailed off, knowing the truth. The money was for drugs.

"So, you're helping him stay sick," I said gently.

She started to cry. "I don't know what else to do."

This is the bind that so many family members find themselves in. They think they have two choices for their loved ones: help in ways that actually enable the addiction, or cut them off completely and let them suffer. Neither feels right. Enabling the addiction doesn't allow them to experience consequences and gets in the way of seeing the need for help. And nobody wants to watch their loved one suffer.

There's a third option: help in ways that actually enable recovery.

That might mean:

• Offering emotional support but not financial support

• Being willing to help them get treatment but not willing to solve the problems their addiction creates

• Setting clear boundaries about what behaviors you will and won't accept

• Taking care of your own well-being first

• When they start to fall, let them experience the consequences of their choices

• Learn about addiction and recovery so you can respond effectively

Breaking the cycle of enabling the disease of addiction isn't easy. It often feels cruel in the short term. But in the long term, it's the most loving thing you can do—both for your addicted loved one and for yourself.

Setting Boundaries That Actually Work

Boundaries are essential in family recovery. But there's a lot of misunderstanding about what boundaries actually are.

Boundaries aren't about controlling someone else's behavior. They're about deciding what you will and won't accept in your life, and then taking action to protect yourself accordingly.

A boundary isn't saying, "You can't drink anymore." It's saying, "I won't be around you when you're drinking."

A boundary isn't saying, "You have to go to rehab." It's saying, "I won't continue to support you financially unless you're actively working on recovery."

A boundary isn't saying, "You can't talk to me that way." It's saying, "If you speak to me disrespectfully, I will end the conversation."

The difference might seem subtle, but it's crucial. Boundaries focus on your behavior, not theirs. They're about what you will do, not what you expect them to do.

And here's the thing about boundaries: they only work if you enforce them consistently.

A boundary that you set and then immediately break just shows the other person that you don't mean what you say.

I worked with a couple once where the wife had set a boundary with her alcoholic husband: if he came home drunk again, she would take the kids and stay with her sister.

One night, he came home clearly intoxicated. She packed a bag, got the kids in the car... and then he started crying, promising it wouldn't happen again, saying he couldn't bear to be without them.

She stayed, breaking her own boundary.

The next day, she was furious with herself. "I failed," she told me.

"You didn't fail," I said. "You learned something. You learned that when he gets emotional, your boundary wavers. Now you can prepare for that next time."

Setting and maintaining boundaries is a skill. It takes practice. It takes support. And sometimes it takes trial and error to find the boundaries that actually work for you.

But it's worth the effort. Because boundaries aren't just about protecting yourself from harmful behavior. They're about creating space for health, growth, and genuine connection.

In a family affected by addiction, good boundaries can be the difference between drowning together and finding a way to shore—even if you don't all get there at the same time.

When to Help and When to Let Go

One of the hardest questions for family members is: When do I keep trying to help, and when do I need to let go?

There's no one-size-fits-all answer to this. It depends on the situation, the relationship, the resources available, and many other factors.

But there are some guiding principles that can help you navigate this difficult territory.

First, consider what kind of help you're offering. Is it help that genuinely supports recovery, or help that inadvertently enables addiction? If you're not sure, ask yourself: If they weren't actively working on recovery, would I still be offering this form of help?

For instance, I generally tell families that paying for good medical insurance is something I would never discourage. Because if they don't have insurance and they need treatment, you're going to end up paying more for it anyway. But paying their rent, their car note, their phone bill? That's different. That's helping them avoid the natural consequences of their addiction, which often keeps them from hitting the bottom they may need to help them make a change. For those who think a phone is important for communication, I'd say that's fine but only a simple flip-phone will do, they don't need the newest iPhone or Android smartphone.

Second, consider the impact on your own well-being. Are you sacrificing your own health, financial security, or emotional stability to help them? If so, that's not sustainable. You can't pour from an empty cup.

I know people who have bankrupted themselves trying to save an addicted loved one. I know people who have developed serious health problems from the stress of constant crisis. I know people who have neglected their other relationships, their work, their own needs in the service of "helping."

That's not helping. That's trying to control and manipulate. And it doesn't serve anyone in the long run.

Third, consider whether your help is actually being received as help. If you're offering treatment options and they're refusing, if you're setting boundaries and they're ignoring them, if you're trying to have honest conversations and they're shutting you down—then your "help" isn't actually helping.

Sometimes the most helpful thing you can do is step back and let the natural consequences unfold. Not out of anger or punishment, but out of respect for their autonomy and their journey.

I've seen families who have had to say to an addicted loved one: "We love you, but we can't watch you destroy yourself anymore. When you're ready to get help, we'll be here. But until then, we need to create some distance."

That's not abandonment. That's recognizing limits—both yours and theirs.

It's also not a one-and-done decision. The balance between helping and letting go can shift over time, depending on what's happening with your loved one's addiction and recovery, what resources are available, and what you're capable of giving.

The key is to keep checking in with yourself, to stay connected to your own values and well-being, and to make decisions from a place of love and clarity rather than fear and obligation.

And remember, you don't have to figure this out alone. There are support groups, therapists, coaches, and others who specialize in helping families navigate these impossible-feeling choices. Reach out. You deserve support too.

Finding Your Own Recovery

If you're reading this as a family member of someone struggling with addiction, I want you to hear something important: You deserve recovery too.

Not just for their sake. For yours.

Your life, your well-being, your joy matters—regardless of whether your loved one ever gets clean.

That can be a hard pill to swallow. We want to believe that if we just love enough, try enough, sacrifice enough, we can save them. And sometimes, our efforts do help. But ultimately, their recovery is their responsibility. Not yours.

Your responsibility is to yourself. To your own healing. To build a life that's worth living, whether they choose recovery or not.

That might sound selfish at first. It's not. It's self-care. And it's actually the best thing you can do for your addicted loved one too.

Because when you start focusing on your own recovery, you naturally stop enabling. You naturally set better boundaries. You naturally create space for them to face the consequences of their choices. And sometimes, that's exactly what they need to decide to change.

"When the family changes it forces the addict to change" - Bob Smith

What does recovery look like for family members? It depends on the person, but it might include:

• Attending Families Anonymous (FA), National Alliance on Mental Health (NAMI), Crisis Text Line, Resilience Project, Hope Not Handcuffs, The Addict's Parents United (APU), Nar-Anon, Gam-Anon or other support groups for families.

• Working with a therapist who understands addiction and family dynamics.

• Learning about addiction so you can separate the person from the disease.

• Setting and maintaining healthy boundaries.

• Reconnecting with your own needs, interests, and joy.

• Building a support system of people who understand what you're going through.

• Practicing self-care in ways that replenish you.

This kind of recovery isn't a luxury or an afterthought. It's a necessity. Because addiction affects the whole family, and recovery must too.

I've seen families transformed when even one member commits to their own recovery—regardless of what the addicted person chooses to do. I've seen spouses find peace, parents find joy, children find stability, all because they decided their own well-being mattered too.

That doesn't mean they stop caring about their addicted loved one. It means they also started caring about themselves. And from that place of balance and health, they're actually able to be more authentically supportive—not from a place of fear, control, or obligation, but from a place of love, clarity, and choice.

That's real recovery. For everyone. Same as when the oxygen masks drop during a flight emergency. So now you know what they mean when they say when the oxygen mask comes down, you place it on yourself first, allowing for survival of all.

Reflection & Practice

If you're a family member of someone struggling with addiction, take some time to reflect on your own journey:

1. How has your loved one's addiction affected you—emotionally, physically, financially, spiritually?

2. What patterns have you developed to cope with the addiction? Which of these are serving you, and which might be keeping you stuck?

3. What would recovery look like for you? Not for them, but for you?

4. What's one small step you could take today toward your own healing?

If you're the person in recovery, consider your family's experience:

1. How has your addiction affected the people you love? Try to see it from their perspective.

2. What patterns might they have developed in response to your addiction? How might they need to heal too?

3. How can you support their recovery while staying focused on your own?

4. What's one conversation you might need to have—when the time is right—to begin healing your family

relationships?

Remember, recovery doesn't happen in isolation. It happens in community. It happens in relationship. It happens when we recognize that we're all in this together—even when we have to walk different paths to find our way home.

Epilogue:
Fasting Forward:
Embracing Imperfection on My 100-Day Journey to Clarity and Health

Throughout history, the way humans have interacted with food has evolved dramatically. Primitive man was a hunter-gatherer who relied on instincts, strength, and endurance to secure meals. This process was arduous and required significant energy, often taking several attempts over days to catch food. Once successful, primitive humans would gorge themselves, consuming as much as they could in a short period. The lack of refrigeration and food storage meant they had to maximize their intake. They were always vigilant against predators who might steal their hard-earned meals, perpetually uncertain about when they would find their next source of sustenance. This lifestyle naturally set the stage for fasting; eating was not a regular occurrence but rather a feast-or-famine existence.

As society advanced and became industrialized, food production and storage transformed. The creation of three meals a day became a cultural norm, moving away from the instinctual eating patterns of our ancestors. Today, our diets are often filled with processed foods, leading to a constant snacking culture reminiscent of cattle grazing throughout the day. This shift has fundamentally altered our relationship with food, distancing us from the natural fasting rhythms that once characterized our existence.

The modern understanding of fasting reveals that it aligns more closely with our evolutionary biology. Research indicates that fasting can promote various health benefits, including weight loss, improved metabolic health, and increased mental clarity. During fasting, the body undergoes significant metabolic changes; as insulin levels drop, the body shifts from using glucose for energy to utilizing fat stores, a process known as ketosis. This metabolic adaptation can enhance brain function and lead to mental clarity as the brain begins to use ketones, a more efficient fuel source.

While weight loss is often a common reason to fast, it's definitely not the only benefit. In addition to improving metabolic health and mental clarity, fasting can improve metabolic health, enhance mental clarity, support immune function, and promote cellular repair. Across cultures, people fast for spiritual or religious reasons, emphasizing personal growth and mindfulness. For example, during Ramadan, Muslims fast from dawn to sunset, while Jews observe Yom Kippur as a time for reflection and repentance through fasting. Hinduism, Buddhism, and various indigenous cultures also have their own unique fasting traditions.

The significance of fasting stretches beyond personal health; it serves as a reminder of the deep-seated connection between our bodies and the natural world. In a time when convenience often takes precedence over mindful consumption, fasting encourages us to listen to our bodies' signals and respect the rhythms of hunger and satiety. It invites us to cultivate a more intentional approach to eating, fostering a deeper appreciation for the nourishment we derive from food and the joy of shared meals.

Now, let's talk about some of the misconceptions surrounding fasting. Many people think fasting is just another word for starvation, believing it's harmful and leads to malnutrition. In reality, fasting is a safe practice that has been used for centuries for health and spiritual reasons. Others worry that it will lead to muscle loss or slow their metabolism, but here's the truth: short-term fasting can actually boost metabolism and help preserve muscle when paired with regular exercise.

My personal journey of fasting began with a challenge to complete a 100-hour fast. Initially skeptical, I agreed to participate after witnessing a friend's determination. The first few hours were manageable; I focused on staying hydrated with carbonated mineral water and engaging in a daily Ethiopian coffee ceremony. As I progressed into the fast, I experienced various physical and emotional responses that provided insights into the fasting process.

At around 36 hours in, I began to feel the effects of fasting. I experienced a partial headache and mental cloudiness, which is common as the body adjusts to a lack of food. However, as I continued, I noticed shifts in my mental state. I felt moments of heightened awareness and increased sensitivity, often described in fasting literature as a result of the body releasing stored energy.

By the time I reached 58 hours, I felt an exhilarating sense of physical pleasure during meditation, accompanied by a buzz of energy that made me feel connected and grateful. These sensations can often be attributed to the release of endorphins and dopamine, which can reset the brain's reward system, leading to increased motivation and focus.

Fasting also fosters significant changes in metabolic health. Research shows that fasting can rejuvenate the immune system, promote autophagy—the body's process of cleaning out damaged cells—and enhance insulin sensitivity. These physiological changes reinforce the idea that fasting is not just a means of weight loss but a beneficial practice for overall health and longevity.

Throughout my fast, I remained mindful of my emotional responses and how they correlated with my food intake. I realized that my dietary choices significantly impacted my mood and mental clarity, providing a powerful insight into how food affects not only physical health but emotional well-being.

As I approached the end of my fast, I felt a sense of accomplishment and clarity. After breaking my fast with nourishing foods, I noticed a remarkable change in my energy levels and mood. Although I had just lost 10 pounds, six hours after completing the fast I engaged in an intense workout on my CLMBR machine. I was able to climb 10,000 feet and clocked myself at 90 minutes—my longest climb ever in distance and time that demonstrated my body's resilience.

This experience reinforced the belief that fasting is not simply an exercise in deprivation, but a transformative journey that reconnects us with our primal instincts and nature.

However, my journey didn't stop there. Just five days after completing my 100-hour fast, I attempted a 7-day fast. I thought I could build on my previous success, but I quickly learned that I was still a work in progress. Thirteen hours into the new fast, I felt tired and drained. It became clear that my body needed more time to recover from the last challenge. At 38 hours, I experienced a throbbing in my temples and was acutely aware of my heartbeat. I realized that my body was signaling me to slow down, reminding me that sometimes, "enough is enough."

I shared these feelings with the five people I had gathered to fast with me, and their varied responses helped me see that it's okay to listen to my body. Ending the fast after 48 hours felt like I was letting the group down, but I was reminded of that earlier chapter in this book about "enough is enough." I still have lessons to learn, and I don't always follow my own advice.

What I'm starting to understand is that my 100-hour fast was a significant accomplishment, and more isn't always better. This realization has been humbling, showing me that I still have work to do in my recovery and personal growth. Also, I learned that as a result of my fast I went down to less than 12% body fat, and at that level extended fasts are not recommended, so ending the second fast when I did was the right decision for me.

In conclusion, my journey of fasting has allowed me to reflect on the ancient practices of our ancestors and how they relate to our current lifestyles. Embracing fasting as a regular part of life can help reestablish a healthier relationship with food, leading to improved mental clarity, emotional stability, and overall well-being. As we move forward in a world filled with convenience and processed foods, returning to the natural rhythms of fasting may be the key to achieving a balanced and healthy life. By reconnecting with these fundamental practices, we not only honor our ancestors but also pave the way for a healthier future for ourselves and generations to come.

About the Author

Michael A. Herbert is an addiction counselor, interventionist, and recovery strategist with over 35 years of experience walking alongside individuals and families through the challenges of addiction and the journey of recovery. Known for his no-nonsense honesty, grounded wisdom, and deep compassion, Michael has worked in treatment centers, clinical settings, correctional institutions, and private practice.

Michael's own recovery journey began on a cold night in Hartford, Connecticut, when he found himself staring at his reflection in a storefront window. That moment of brutal honesty became the foundation for over three decades of recovery. It was the beginning of a lifetime dedicated to helping others find their own path to healing.

What sets Michael apart is his willingness to live recovery out loud. He's climbed mountains on four continents, run ultramarathons through the Sahara Desert, fed wild hyenas in Ethiopia, and lived with the Tarahumara Indians in Mexico.

As the founder of African Hopeful Horizons, a nonprofit organization, Michael has transformed education in rural Ethiopia. What began as a simple promise to bring school supplies to a village whose school had been destroyed by a dust storm has grown into a comprehensive program. It now provides educational materials for three schools, builds sustainable lunch programs through chicken farming, and gives

136 students access to proper desks, supplies, and learning environments.

Michael's approach to recovery is refreshingly practical and deeply personal. He offers tools, stories, and real talk that speak directly to anyone ready to face their truth, take ownership of their healing, and stay in the work. His philosophy is built on five core values: integrity, creativity, perseverance, trust, and humility.

Throughout his career, Michael has worked with CEOs and janitors, doctors and day laborers, parents and parolees. His clients range from high-profile professionals to everyday people who've decided they're tired of living a life that doesn't feel like their own.

Michael is also a world traveler, beekeeper, athlete, and mentor. Whether he's running through the desert, climbing an active volcano, or sitting quietly with a client in his office, he brings the same energy. Curiosity, courage, and an unshakable belief that change is possible.

Through his writing, coaching, and speaking, Michael helps people take responsibility for their healing and build lives rooted in integrity, curiosity, and lasting change.

CONTINUE YOUR JOURNEY

Recovery is a journey, not a destination. If the stories and insights in this book resonated with you, this is just the beginning.

CONNECT WITH MICHAEL

Visit www.coachmichaelherbert.com or email michael@coachmichaelherbert.com to access resources designed to complement what you've learned.

Free Resources:

Recovery assessments to help you understand where you are in your journey

Downloadable worksheets for each of the five core values

Audio meditations and reflection exercises

Monthly blog posts with new insights and practical tools

Paid Programs:

One-on-one recovery coaching sessions with Michael

Group coaching programs for individuals and families

Intensive weekend workshops focused on building sustainable recovery

Adventure-based recovery experiences

Family recovery programs that address the whole system

FOR FAMILIES AND LOVED ONES

Recovery affects everyone in the family system. If you're the spouse, parent, child, or friend of someone struggling with addiction, you need support too. Visit the website to learn about family recovery coaching, support groups, and tools for setting healthy boundaries.

SPEAKING AND WORKSHOPS

Michael is available for speaking engagements, corporate workshops, and treatment center presentations. His talks combine personal storytelling with practical tools, offering audiences both inspiration and actionable strategies.

A PERSONAL MESSAGE FROM MICHAEL

Recovery gave me my life back. But more than that, it gave me a life I never knew was possible. The adventures I've had, the relationships I've built, the work I get to do. None of it would exist without the foundation of recovery.

Your recovery doesn't have to look like mine. Your path might lead to mountains or museums, boardrooms or bakeries, quiet contemplation or loud celebration. What matters is that it's authentically yours.

The tools in this book work. The five core values provide a foundation that can support any kind of life you want to build. But knowing about them isn't enough. You have to live them, practice them, and adjust them to fit your unique circumstances.

That's where ongoing support comes in. Recovery isn't a solo project. It's something you build in community, with guidance, and over time. The resources on my website are designed to help you take what you've learned here and apply it to your real life, your real challenges, your real dreams.

Whether you're just starting out, feeling stuck in the middle, or looking to deepen a recovery you've already begun, there's something there for you.

I've had the privilege of walking alongside thousands of people as they've built lives they never thought possible. Some have climbed literal mountains. Others have climbed metaphorical ones. All have discovered that recovery isn't about getting your old life back. It's about creating a new one.

Your recovery matters. Your story matters. Your life matters.

Visit www.coachmichaelherbert.com or email michael@coachmichaelherbert.com today and take the next step in your journey.

Remember, this is your life. This is your recovery. Let's build something worth staying for.

For immediate support or crisis intervention, contact your local emergency services or call the National Suicide Prevention Lifeline at 988. If you're struggling with substance use, call SAMHSA's National Helpline at 1-800-662-HELP (4357) for free, confidential treatment referrals and information.

www.ingramcontent.com/pod-product-compliance
Lightning Source LLC
Chambersburg PA
CBHW030847090426
42737CB00009B/1127